BREAKING THE CHAIN
OF DISEASE

BREAKING THE CHAIN OF DISEASE

RICHARD F. DEROSE

iUniverse, Inc.
Bloomington

Breaking the Chain of Disease

iUniverse books may be ordered through booksellers or by contacting:

iUniverse
1663 Liberty Drive
Bloomington, IN 47403
www.iuniverse.com
1-800-Authors (1-800-288-4677)

Because of the dynamic nature of the Internet, any web addresses or links contained in this book may have changed since publication and may no longer be valid. The views expressed in this work are solely those of the author and do not necessarily reflect the views of the publisher, and the publisher hereby disclaims any responsibility for them.

Any people depicted in stock imagery provided by Thinkstock are models, and such images are being used for illustrative purposes only.

Certain stock imagery © Thinkstock.

ISBN: 978-1-4620-8256-8 (sc)
ISBN: 978-1-4620-8255-1 (e)
ISBN: 978-1-4620-8254-4 (dj)

Printed in the United States of America

iUniverse rev. date: 1/5/2012

Cover design by Dan Kugle

To my wife, Deirdre, for her continual encouragement unwavering support, and endearing love, which gave me the strength to pursue my dream.

The only sure cure for all disease is death

Contents

PREFACE

The timing for writing this book is crucial because of alarming current events as they relate to disease worldwide.

First, let me make it perfectly clear that I am neither a professional writer nor a medical officer. However, my studies and training are directly related to epidemiology, which is the study of epidemics and pandemics. An Epidemic is when a disease affects many people at the same time and spreads from person to person in a locality where the disease is not permanently prevalent. In comparison, a Pandemic occurs over a wide geographic area and affects an exceptionally high proportion of the population.

If for any reason my writing technique disappoints or offends you in any way, I apologize. However, the information you hold in your hands has been verified for clarity, content, and accuracy by individuals in many different research arenas. None of the following information is based on speculation or theory.

The contents of *Breaking the Chain of Disease* are not aimed at changing your feelings, beliefs, or thought patterns. As you read, you'll be taken on a completely different journey as it relates to infectious diseases. If you have never attended one of my training seminars, let me explain that my goal has always been to help my audience identify the potential risks they may be faced with given the environment and contacts they are routinely exposed to.

Forget what you've heard, learned, or studied. What you are about to read will enlighten you and stir your emotions and curiosity, as well as give you the resolution to live a disease-free life.

Ignorance is not bliss as it relates to infectious diseases. What you don't know will eventually harm you. You need to take action, open your arms, and embrace the principles I discuss in this book. You will then gain the awareness and, most importantly, have the tools and resources to break the chain of disease.

Infectious diseases are in evolutionary overdrive. We discover a new disease that we have never seen before every twenty minutes every day somewhere in the world, as reported by the Center for Disease Control and Prevention, located in Atlanta, Georgia.

In this era of modern science and medical breakthroughs, why are we still in the position of losing control of diseases throughout the world?

Scientists have collaborated in the development of new drugs and medical management procedures to combat diseases that impact every person in every Continent, Country, and City Worldwide. These efforts continue to fail. One would think, given the advancements in science over the last fifty years, which has progressed more than the previous five hundred years, we would have more control over the increasing impact that infectious diseases have on us as human beings. The World Health Organization, United Nations, National Institute of Health, and the Center for Disease Control and Prevention all continue to mislead and misrepresent their mission statements to those they have been commissioned to protect.

Because of genetic engineering, we have the ability to eradicate hundreds of diseases. Those entities capable of doing so, however, choose not to because if you don't get sick, there are no profits for them. I am not referring to cancers, diabetes, or heart and lung conditions. The diseases I specifically address in this book are related only to microbes.

The Food and Drug Administration (FDA) has collaborated with the most powerful and profitable pharmaceutical companies to develop drugs, vaccines, and other medicines that repeatedly fail or have significant life-threatening side effects. In 2010, the FDA received thousands of applications for new drugs and antibiotics, of which only seventy were approved to be used by the general public. The pharmaceutical companies develop these products, and then apply to the FDA for approval. The fact that the FDA approved only seventy such medicines would show that the majority of them fail or have bad side effects.

The pharmaceutical companies pick and choose the drugs they believe will be the most profitable, not necessarily the most effective or safest. The average cost for an agency's stamp of approval for such drugs is in the range of 60 to 100 million dollars, and development takes on average five years of research. These costs are passed down to us, the consumers, in exorbitant fees. It is a known fact according to the Internal Revenue Service's public records that pharmaceutical companies make billions—excuse me, *trillions*—of dollars a year worldwide on medical conditions they now define as a disease. What is most startling to me is that the presidents and CEOs of these major pharmaceutical companies sit on the same steering and approval committees that sanction their drugs.

United States Government Health Agencies, such as Medicare and Medi-Cal estimate the annual cost of medical care for treating infectious diseases in the United States alone is 120 billion dollars. Given this fact and the forecasted epidemics and pandemics on the horizon, this amount can only increase. The reason why the human race shouldn't be as sick as we are today is directly related to greed in the pharmaceutical industry.

The United States Federal Government passed legislation in September 2009 authored by Kathleen Swendiman that gave power to the Health and Human Resources Department, with the backing of federal and state law enforcement agencies, to implement and ensure compliance with mandatory influenza vaccinations. This legislation gave our own government the power to force us, the people, to submit at "gunpoint" to take vaccines, some of which hadn't yet been tested on humans. Basically, this is legalized murder.

To fully understand the world of disease and its impact on us as human beings, first you must explore the history and future of infectious diseases and their existence in society as a whole. You cannot see, smell, or taste what exists around you every day, but it has all of the components to invade and destroy vital organs and systems in your body that can lead to sickness or death.

Ask yourself this question: Have you ever been sick a day in your life and didn't know where you got it?

Of course, the answer should be yes. This is because our daily routine exposes us to microbes and pathogens every day that we are not aware of. Understand that these microscopic organisms do not discriminate. These disease-causing microbes exist in every environment. They don't care what you do for a living, the color of your skin, whether you're male or female, or what your age or sexual preferences are. They are simply looking for a human host. We human beings are the five-star restaurants that every microbe thrives on. Our bodies contain all of the ingredients they need to survive. We carry both nutrients and cells, everything they need from a human host.

The place where you are reading this book right now, whether it be your home, office, airport, or restaurant, is filled with bacteria, viruses, fungi, and parasites.

If this is true, why don't we get sick every day? Simply put, we have two very important defensive mechanisms, which are your skin and immune system that prevent us from getting sick from the daily contact we have with these microorganisms that exist all around us.

The following information is not designed to change your feelings, beliefs, or thought patterns. That is not my concern, nor is it my training. If you engage in certain behavior, I will clearly explain why you may be at risk. If you decide to change that behavior, you will have reduced the chances of being exposed and, therefore, infected.

There is a saying that there are no guarantees in life. I beg to differ. This book will change the way you approach life, how you interact with others, the places you go, where you choose to eat and exercise, and even where you seek medical treatment. If you apply the principles I discuss in this book, I guarantee you will have the awareness and most importantly the tools and resources to break the chain of disease.

By reading this book, you will learn that there are essential elements that must be present at the time of exposure for any disease to be passed on from one human host to another. There are four elements within that chain of transmission. If you can eliminate just one of those elements, you will not be infected, regardless of the activity you are engaged in.

My wife recently presented me with a perfect analogy to help you better understand this. If you were baking a cake, for instance, and left out just one ingredient, your cooking effort would fail. The cake would not turn out. This is similar to disease. If you eliminate one of the elements in the chain of transmission, I guarantee you that it, too, will fail; you will not become a new human host.

Mainstream medicine has benefited some but failed many. We have alternative approaches through what is referred to as Naturopathic Medicine, unorthodox means of medical care and treatment that is available to everyone in every country. This I will discuss further in chapter 7. Take control of your own health and life. It is possible that you can lead a disease-free life.

My goal is to lead you to such a disease-free life.

CHAPTER 1
EVOLUTION OF DISEASE:
PAST, PRESENT, AND FUTURE

Where do I begin? I suppose from the beginning.

Epidemiology, that is, the research and study of disease, existed well before Christ. In fact, in 30 BC a new and deadly disease emerged and swept through Athens, Greece; still to this day, it remains a mystery. At the same time, war erupted between Athenian and Spartan soldiers, which led refugees and citizens to live on the streets filled with war casualties. Then the social order broke down.

During the next three years, the illness returned twice. Could this type of outbreak happen again today or in the near future, given the unprovoked social violence and modern-day wars occurring in every corner of the world? A great majority of the scientific community believes it will.

The city of Athens lost a third of its population to this mysterious disease. Can you imagine if this were to occur in US cities as large as New York, Chicago, and Los Angeles, or cities overseas such as Tokyo, Sydney, or London? This type of outbreak marked the beginning of modern-day epidemiology.

Disease outbreaks have a long history prior to Influenzas, Hepatitis, HIV/AIDS, Sexually Transmitted diseases (STDs), and other emergent diseases of the modern era. There appear to be several common determinants on whether new diseases will emerge that will impede human progress.

Examples of these common determinants are open borders, population growth, change in climate and ecosystems, lack of medical care and treatment, human behavior, and political malpractice.

The art of predicting disease emergence is not well-developed. We know, however, that mixtures of these determinants have become more complex. For example, there are more people traveling internationally today then ever before. A disease that typically took weeks, if not months, to spread to other areas of the world now literally can reach the other side of the earth within twenty-four hours.

A businessman visiting China, for instance, could be exposed to an Influenza Virus, such as H1N1 or SARS, and then jump on a plane to North America just hours after exposure. After just forty-eight to seventy-two hours, he has the ability to spread the disease among those he casually comes in contact with, such as business associates and family members and friends.

This increased mobility was clearly linked to the outbreak of the novel illness SARS in 2003, which rapidly spread from Hong Kong to Toronto and all other corners of the globe in less than thirty days. The World Health Organization (WHO) became suspicious when the Prime Minister of China placed a gag order on China's health administrators, media representatives, and most startling United Nations representatives. The sheer lack of concern for human safety unfortunately compromised the ability of scientists around the world to set into motion the steps necessary to eradicate the disease. Once the virus subsided, the final tally of death reached into the thousands. *It was preventable.*

It's well documented that other diseases have spread this way, such as Tuberculosis, Meningitis, and Influenza, to name a few. As we look at epidemiology, or the history of diseases, since the beginning of recorded history, epidemics have always been caused by particular microorganisms or pathogens. Historically, for example, the Black Death, referring to the Bubonic Plague, which killed some 34 million Europeans in the middle of the fourteenth century, was caused by bacteria. A smallpox epidemic afflicted the Aztec Indians of Mexico in the sixteenth century. Smallpox had ravished European communities for centuries, but until the Spanish arrived on the Yucatan Coast in 1519, the disease was unknown in the New World. Historical records indicate that 3.5 million people in Central Mexico died in the first year of this epidemic.

Forensic evidence of these epidemics and pandemics has proven the devastating numbers of deaths inflicted by these outbreaks. What is more sobering is to walk the grave sites in these countries, and you will be overwhelmed by the number of families completely wiped out by disease. A real eye-opener is reading the tombstones, which are a true indicator of the time of death occurring within months of each other.

Dozens of other epidemics have occurred more recently in the seventeenth and eighteenth centuries. Between the years of 1793 through 1798, there was an outbreak of Yellow Fever in the state of Pennsylvania, with the hot zone being the capital, Philadelphia. This outbreak took hundreds of thousands of lives during those years.

Moving forward, during the 1830s, Cholera made its way through Asia and Europe. In fact, French officials attempted to prepare their country in advance of the outbreak. Teams of doctors, nurses, and health inspection officers progressed on the borders and ports. They were assigned to inspect wells, cesspools, and latrines of both public and private buildings. Despite all their efforts, within two weeks there were a thousand cases reported, 80 percent of them fatal.

This was the first time in history that a large-scale emerging epidemic was actually scientifically investigated in real time. Researchers looked at concepts that could have been responsible for the high mortality and morbidity rates, including ages of the victims, sex, occupation, and socioeconomic status. Since then, there have been numerous outbreaks, epidemics, and pandemics throughout the world that have been investigated by utilizing these same tools, skills, and techniques.

Modern epidemiology, considered that of the twentieth century, was not exempt from these catastrophic events. The influenza outbreak of 1918 and 1919 was a perfect example. The death tolls have been estimated between 28 to 40 million people worldwide. Many scientific studies and research indicate that the next hundred-year plague will strike earlier than forecasted. If this event were to occur, estimates put the death toll at 60 to 100 million people around the globe.

Modern medicine has progressed more in the last fifty years than in the previous five hundred years. With antiviral agents, antibiotics, and vaccines available to basically anyone in the world, why do these epidemics still pose a great risk to civilization? It is said that timing is everything in life. Timing unfortunately may be the catapult in which a combination of viruses together will attack the most susceptible victims, namely us, the human race. This particular Influenza Virus, which will be a combination of the Avian, Swine and Human Flu Viruses, will overwhelm our hospitals and medical supply systems. There simply will not be enough vaccines that can be issued fast enough to stall or eradicate this plague. In fact, and I say it as a joke, there wouldn't be enough chicken eggs in the world to develop the amount of vaccines to accommodate every potential taker that is vulnerable to these Influenza Viruses.

If supplies of vaccines were depleted, another option would be genetic engineering. However, the costs to genetically engineer a vaccination or immunization against these types of disease would not be fiscally possible. Other Influenza outbreaks have occurred in North America and other parts of the world in 1977, 1985, and 1999. These most recent outbreaks may be the precursor of what could be the next hundred-year plague.

If we compare this hundred-year plague with all other epidemics and pandemics that exist in the world today, for instance, HIV, Dengue, Tuberculosis, and Hepatitis, it is believed within the scientific and medical communities that this would have the potential to develop into the greatest human plague of the Modern Era.

Consider this: a person is infected with HIV every nine seconds somewhere in the world. In the time it takes to read this sentence, someone has just been infected with the Human Immunodeficiency Virus. HIV is typically more difficult to transmit than other viruses because it requires intimate contact with an infectious carrier, whereas Influenza is airborne. This demonstrates how vulnerable we all are to an airborne virus.

Members of the scientific community are actually going backward in their research. These diseases spread so fast and without any warning that we can't possibly keep up with them. We are further behind now than we were ten years ago in developing new antibiotics, antiviral agents, and vaccines that would create immunity to or treat the illness itself.

History, as you know, is supposed to teach us lessons, but past flu pandemics haven't taught us much as to the future outbreaks that may actually occur. To use a quote from the Associated Press, "bird flu will become a mega killer" or will just make scientists and researchers look like "Chicken Little." Granted, in previous centuries, there were insufficient surveillance systems or modern genetic tools to detect and document viruses as they evolved into killer strains. Even today, we don't have a crystal ball that would grant us the advantage to forecast catastrophic events. Due to the lack of knowledge and documentation of past outbreaks, the medical community is at the mercy of the next mega super flu, hundred-year plague, or next great pandemic.

If we look at the history of epidemiology as it stands concerning some of these epidemics and pandemics we have been discussing, the H1N1 Influenza outbreak doesn't come close in comparison to the lethal flu germs from the past. The 2009 event cannot legitimately be called a pandemic. According to the Center for Disease Control and Prevention, more people die from the annual flu in North America every year (approximately 32,000), than the total global impact of the H1N1 novel virus.

In November 2005, government health officials announced to the public, and I quote from the Bloomberg News Report, that "we are in a race against nature." The U.S. Institute of Medicine indicated in an article for the Mortality and Morbidity Weekly Report, that the bird flu has the potential to kill 1.9 million Americans and could hospitalize 9.9 million.

Given this information, President George Bush unveiled a 7.1-billion-dollar flu plan that could stockpile flu vaccines for early responders. The plan wouldn't take full effect until 2010 at the earliest, which has been delayed indefinitely because the earmarked funds for vaccine development have been redirected to other programs.

Government officials are trying to push through the biggest flu vaccination program in U.S. History for the general populous. This would become an annual flu vaccination campaign involving flu shots for all Americans. It would be a massive program delivering more vaccines than all other vaccines combined. Even if we were to vaccinate only two-thirds of the United States population, it would cost an estimated 2 billion dollars in its first year. Many people do not fall in the high-risk category and would be forced to take a vaccine they don't need. I will discuss that in Chapter 8, "To Vaccinate or Not to Vaccinate (It's Your Decision)."

Even if world governments were to establish funding for these large arsenals of vaccines, we would still have to orchestrate and deploy the vaccines around the world to save possibly millions of lives. Some food for thought: the more virulent the influenza strain, the greater chances for side effects with the shots. New approaches of prevention would be needed to avoid these inevitable complications.

President George Bush's plan was a perfect example of complacency. His directive did not meet its objectives of protecting millions of Americans from a potential Influenza pandemic. The lack of education and awareness at the highest levels plays a major role in the spread of disease. People worldwide deserve better.

Preventable infections all too often are the results of errors in diagnosis and adverse events not detected early enough, which kill hundreds of thousands of Americans as well as millions worldwide each year. Our health-care systems are facing a certain crisis of epidemic proportions. We have unfortunately settled into a state of complacency and a degraded approach to human health and life.

Now that we have an idea of how the history of epidemiology has evolved and what is currently happening in the field of disease, we have to seriously consider the effects of these types of outbreaks in our future. There are many learned medical approaches that can identify and possibly eradicate these diseases using genetic mapping, accounts from historical epidemics, and documented deaths, illnesses, and hospitalizations. It's time we face the new evolution of these microbes and take aggressive actions to prevent the spread of disease.

History can definitely teach us lessons of prevention if we look at it carefully enough, giving us a new and more profound approach in fighting these outbreaks that may have a catastrophic effect impacting society worldwide. World Health Organization leaders have admitted that they have been thrown an epidemic curveball. So, what got us to this point? Is it research that may not be up-to-date? Is it the lack of fiscal responsibility? Is it simply not advancing fast enough with research and treatments? These questions remain unanswered.

There have been numerous milestones with advancements in genetic engineering, which now has been around for more than half a century. So, why is there a lack of better understanding of how these microbes and pathogens continually mutate and infiltrate themselves in living hosts?

The prescription has been written.

We are on the precipice of a global epidemic in regard to blood-borne, food-borne, and airborne disease that we have never seen in the history of epidemiology. There is no argument that strengthening our health-care system and effective care will reduce illness and death among those stricken. Humanitarian aid has the greatest impact of all. Getting to the core of the new evolution of disease and the demographics in which it has impacted will help isolate these outbreaks and prevent them from mutating and spreading to uninfected areas of the globe. When new strains have developed that put us all in harm's way, the scientific and medical communities' ability to control and treat these diseases decreases significantly with every day that passes.

If you haven't figured it out yet, our greatest adversaries are the microbes themselves. A microbe is defined as a minute life-form that is the cause of all disease. As you move forward in this book, you will see that you have complete control over your own destiny, your own life and health. There is a saying I mention consistently in my public seminars: "If you were to wait for your employer, government agencies, health-care provider, or even your own private physician to protect you, you'll be waiting forever."

For years, even I thought these entities were our greatest adversaries, but as I continued my research, I found it starts with the microbe—a tiny organism that you may not see, smell, or taste, but that exists all around you in every environment. Many of these microbes have been identified and given names, such as HIV/AIDS, Hepatitis, Tuberculosis, Polio, MRSA, and Sexually Transmitted Disease (STD), such as Herpes.

What many of you may not be aware of is that these original microbes, whether virus, bacterium, fungus, or parasite, change in order to adapt to new living environments and the human host as well. For example, HIV has type 1 and type 2. Recently through research, we have discovered six new types of HIV in the world. Each type has twenty-eight to thirty-two different strains to it, and each strain can mutate four times to the nine-thousandth power, which gives it an infinite number of mutations. HIV is different in every single person's body. That is why some carriers of this disease succumb to the disease process within months of acquiring it and others can live years without showing any symptoms.

Tuberculosis has evolved into a significant respiratory ailment. Although the disease can be diagnosed with a simple skin test, it has changed also, similar to HIV, by developing new strains that make it resistant to current antibacterial treatments. The formal terms are MDR-TB and XDR-TB, both of which carry the unique factor of being multidrug resistant, including in some cases chemotherapy and radiation. In fact, on rare occasions, we cannot eliminate its active presence in the human host.

According to the World Health Association it is estimated that one third of the world's population is a carrier of tuberculosis and nearly 9 million persons develop TB disease. From 1985 through 1992, the United States was confronted with an unprecedented TB resurgence. During this resurgence along came MDR-TB, which is defined as multidrug-resistant TB. Shortly after the discovery of MDR-TB emerged XDR-TB, this means extreme drug-resistant TB.

XDR-TB has been identified in all regions of the world, including the United States. To give you an idea of the financial impact this one disease has on one patient and the medical systems as a whole, the average cost of hospitalization, antibiotic therapy, follow-up treatment, and testing equates to hundreds of thousands of dollars per patient. If XDR-TB were to develop into a full-scale epidemic, the health-care system could not handle the fiscal impact.

The U.S. Government has created a task force to combat a potential outbreak of this disease here in our homeland. The components that have been addressed and implemented are similar to those for a flu epidemic: rapid testing of all citizens, increasing the availability and access to the vaccine, voluntary isolation, mandatory quarantine, and commandeering military sites as makeshift hospitals for treatment. Travel restrictions would be put in place, with no International travel to or from epidemic or pandemic regions of the world.

This plan was put into use a few years back when a passenger boarded a plane heading to the United States against doctor's orders. Upon arrival, the person was immediately apprehended by government officials, placed in isolation, and treated for active TB. Fortunately, this particular individual was not a carrier of the drug-resistant strain. Once the symptoms went away, the patient was no longer considered a health risk to others and was released. Other passengers exposed to him during the flight had to be contacted by the health authorities for questioning and testing.

Hepatitis for years has been considered to have three common types: A, B, and C. Medical researchers worldwide, with the endorsement and confirmation of the World Health Organization (WHO), National Institutes of Health (NIH), Centers for Disease Control and Prevention (CDC), and *The Journal of American Medical Association*, have identified hepatitis types D through H which was discovered in 1977. The New England Journal of Medicine published and article that same year confirming these discoveries.

Polio, a disease that we believed had been eradicated from the face of the earth, has now evolved, and scientists and medical specialists around the world are fearful we may have to revaccinate the entire world's population within the next decade.

Sexually transmitted diseases (STD), such as Herpes, are at the highest rates we have ever seen in history. Also, we have seen a significant increase in cases reported of Syphilis, Gonorrhea, Chlamydia, and the Human Papillon Virus (HPV).

Skin infections—referred to as flesh-eating diseases—are also on the rise. For instance, Methicillin-Resistant s\Staphylococcal Aureus (MRSA) is at its highest level ever, with approximately 142,000 cases reported by the CDC, leading to 18,650 deaths in the United States in 2008. Recently a new type of staph infection has evolved, called Vancomycin Intermediate/Resistant Staphlococcus aureus (VISA), just as in the credit card.

"And yes, it is accepted all over the world."

The Centers for Disease Control and Prevention (CDC) and other reputable health organizations have concluded that individual interventions or specific combinations of interventions appropriate to health-care facilities may not eradicate Staph. All of these diseases are related to microbial enemies. What new offspring will develop in the future? There is no answer to this question; we must live it out to see the outcome.

CHAPTER 2
SOCIAL MICROBE FACTORIES

One would think, given everything I know and have learned through formal education about infectious diseases, that I would never step foot out of my own home—that I would isolate myself from the outside world, like a man in a bubble. That, however, is unrealistic and not necessary. In fact, just the opposite is true, which is exactly why I've chosen this journey to help others understand the world that we live in, which at times may appear on the surface to be dangerous but is mainly harmless. As I discussed in the first chapter, these microbes, such as bacteria, have been around since the beginning of time. There is no argument that these microscopic enemies have changed over time and have taken many lives. What is more concerning is that these same microbes can destroy our allies, good germs.

If I were to dissect your daily routine, I could identify numerous situations that could compromise your good health and put you in harm's way. Why, then, don't we get sick every day? Such questions will be addressed throughout this book. My goal is to help you help yourself. This can be achieved by eliminating any misconceptions or phobias you have about disease.

Recently, I was watching a newscast about an outbreak of a food-borne disease called Salmonella, which was linked back to a source of ground turkey meat. The media jumped all over this from every angle to the point of almost glamorizing its existence like we would the next American Idol or Biggest Loser. These types of outbreaks are a result of unhealthy working conditions and practices and a breakdown in the processing operations, refrigeration, transportation, and shelving of perishable items we put in our bodies every day. Food-borne illnesses account for approximately 76 million cases per year in the United States, leading to 325,000 hospitalizations and 5000 deaths, according to the World Health Organization in an article date April 2007.

Typically when I'm deciding which restaurant to eat at, it's usually from a trusted recommendation from a friend or family member. My decision is rarely made after reading the *big* letter rating that has been posted by the health department on the front window. If the food is good and the pricing reasonable, they will most likely get a return visit from me. When I eat in an establishment other than my own kitchen, I am constantly (some would say obsessively) checking out the utensils, the servers, and the servers' work practices. Careful consideration to eat at certain establishments is based on the restaurants' specialties. I wouldn't order fish in a burger joint, nor would I go to a fish and chips restaurant and order a tasty filet mignon. All of this is to give me a little sense of security and safety.

Even the most educated eye can miss things, however, as can be validated by the following situation. One afternoon I was eating at a food chain whose name I will keep confidential for disclaimer reasons. They had what appeared to be a very large soup and salad bar, with numerous condiments, dressings, and produce. Ahh! What could be better on a warm summer day than a nice crisp, cold, fresh, build-your-own salad? After serving myself and returning to my booth, where my clients were waiting for their orders from the invisible kitchen in the back, I noticed a woman take the serving spoon out of the potato salad and place it in her mouth to see how it tasted. To my surprise, she then placed that same utensil back into the salad, covered with her saliva, mucous, sputum, and who knows what other bodily secretions that were in her mouth. Being the Good Samaritan that I am, I immediately caught the attention of the manager and told him what I had just witnessed. Did the action of replacing the same spoon back in the salad pose a threat to my health and that of other, unsuspecting patrons? Of course, the answer is without a doubt, *yes*. In fact, the mouth and its secretions harbor more disease than even your rectum (feces). My daughter would say, "(TMI), to much information".

Clinical research and testing has proven the mouth to be a means of transmission of disease. The mouth and its secretions is considered the most infectious part of the body. In fact, it's more infectious than the rectum and its secretions. Feces contain everything your system doesn't need, want, and is able to get rid of through these secretions. According to my own research at the University of Irvine, California, the mouth contains a hundred times more infectious disease-causing agents than the rectum. Then, you wonder why you caught a disease such as Hepatitis, Herpes, Colds, or the Flu. Well, what part of other people's body do you usually come in contact with, the mouth or the rectum? Maybe you should keep that answer private, but never overlook the risk of that kind of contact. Enough with the salad bar story.

Going back to the subject of food-related illnesses, one of the worst side effects short of death would be food poisoning. I have personally experienced this a few times in my life. I chalk it up to the fact that my consulting business was awarded numerous contracts with law enforcement departments and I felt obligated to eat the food prepared within the prison facilities by the inmates, despite many warnings from the officers. Let me just for a moment share with you the physical pain that followed my consumption of one such wonderful meal. After all, the prisoners were treating me like a dignitary. It would have been extremely rude not to eat the food prepared by these chefs. Let me just say, to this day, I have yet to identify which course of food led to what I considered to be my "near-death" experience.

It began about an hour into my afternoon lecture, when I started to experience small stomach cramps. Just minutes later, the cramping became more severe. What followed next is typical with this type of poisoning—the daunting feeling of nausea. Now we all know what follows nausea. You're correct if you guessed vomiting. For your educated guess and as Jim Carey said in the movie, Liar Liar "*Ding, ding, ding,* what to do we have for her Johnny, *It's a new suit.*" Fortunately for me, I was close to a bathroom. After revisiting my lunch for the third time, I began to feel better until I decided to stand up. You see, at this point, your body is actually doing what is necessary to get rid of the toxin or poison that has invaded your gastrointestinal tract. Suddenly, in walked one of my students. The officer asked me if I needed help, and all I could muster in words was that I needed a priest for an exorcism. The nurse was called from the infirmary. She placed me in a wheelchair to assist me back to the medical clinic for IV Fluids; I trailed evidence of my experience the entire way. I felt at this moment nothing but pain and sincere sympathy for the janitorial staff that had to remove my lunch from the walkway.

Cases like mine happen so often and frequently with life-threatening consequences that all Health Departments, along with the Food and Drug Administration, have created and implemented strict code requirements for all restaurants, salad bars, and buffet displays. One obvious requirement is that any opened, exposed food must be shielded to block a direct hit from a cough or sneeze from a customer's mouth or nose into the food on display. I usually refer to these barriers as snot guards. For larger displays of food, it is required that establishments install transparent plastic or glass shields angled to prevent oral secretions from coming in contact with the food. If there is no evidence of these types of guards, then the establishments are out of compliance and could be written up with corrective actions and fined by the Health Department. A separate utensil with a handle is required for each food item. Remember my own salad bar experience. No customer is ever allowed to touch the food with his or her hands or mouth. If you witness this, report it to your server or a manager ASAP.

Something that often goes overlooked and generally is the customer's fault is using a serving spoon then touching their dirty plate. A clean setup should always be used. Proper food temperature is critical to kill any disease-causing microbes in food. Cold foods should be displayed on ice or buried in ice and hot food under heat lamps. *Do not* trust chafing dishes for long-term heating (longer than two hours). Generally you will see chafing dishes at temporary food displays. Finally, the employees must be trained and implement required hygiene practices, such as regular hand washing and monitoring and maintaining fresh food products and replenishing them to the proper food temperatures using approved food thermometers.

If you haven't figured it out yet, we live in a germ-filled world. These microbes not only occupy the places where we eat, but also occupy places that make us happy enjoying the freedoms we have in life, such as the theater, amusement parks, museums, cruise ships, planes, trains, beaches, water parks, wet decks, and spray pads. Shared places, such as our homes, churches, and schools, contain the same levels of microorganisms similar to most public places. These places, which are supposed to be the happiest places on earth, are a microbe's five-star hotel.

Did you ever wonder how safe or hygienically sound public water parks are for our kids? As I observed my children playing with other kids in this fun H2O facility, I questioned could harmful germs exist in this water park? Was that yellow or slightly pea green-colored water really as clean as they advertised? There are many regulations and compliance standards these parks are legally responsible to implement in their facilities. Are these facilities maintaining the appropriate chemical levels for the volume of water to kill off the parasites, spores, bacteria, or viruses that are occupying and sharing the same space as your unsuspecting child? Has the water temperature been adjusted to ensure that these microscopic organisms cannot survive due to the heat indexes that can potentially destroy them? Are the filtration devices installed *properly* to ensure these enemies are no longer being recycled back to your child for a second go-around? The more times you are exposed to these pathogens and the longer you're in that environment, the greater the chances you have of becoming infected. Then you wonder how your child developed pinkeye, a skin condition, or flu-like symptoms. Well, I just told you how.

The CDC reports that each year these types of unnecessary exposures occur approximately thirty to forty thousand times, leading to illness, hospitalization, and even death, all of which is preventable. A case in point: The CDC reported that an outbreak in 1999 of a diarrheal illness affected 44 percent of patrons out of 4800 who visited a new local wet deck in Beachside Park. Officials from the health department determined after an investigation that the water from the wet deck plus human secretions draining into an underground reservoir for recirculation was the culprit. This practice, inadequate chlorination, and no filtration systems were the root causes for the outbreak. Again, this could have been prevented. We also cannot forget that human error can often be blamed for these types of outbreaks. In this case, the maintenance personnel had overlooked critical decontamination procedures, such as filling the chlorine tablet erosion feeder; filling it was "two weeks overdue."

A similar case was reported by the CDC in 2005, which envolved a vector-borne enteric disease that was discovered at Seneca Lake State Water Park, New York. During the summer, an outbreak of cryptosporidiosis infected 1700 people, with 425 confirmed lab cases.

The disease was traced to the water tanks of the 11,000-square-foot wet deck. Sanitation practices were again overlooked and identified as the direct cause for the outbreak. Representatives of the New York State Health Department said in their report of findings, this could have been avoided.

If you use a water source at home or in your community, you should take on the added responsibility of assuring that these types of practices are not overlooked. Never assume that the person who is responsible for assuring your safety and that of anyone else utilizing these pools, jacuzzis, and many other water source designs is doing his or her job efficiently.

I don't want myself or my child to be the first documented case of disease, do you?

Everyone attending these parks should be more observant of these environments to ensure personal safety and that of their child or children. This practice doesn't just apply to the hygienic procedures that have been put into action by the facility, but just as important not to knowingly allow yourself or others to participate when ill, regardless of how saddened they may feel. If your child, for instance, has an obvious cold, flu, or other respiratory problem, *keep him or her home.*

Exposing a child and his or her illness to others simply spreads it to an innocent victim. In addition, the carrier's immune system is compromised or weakened, because of the secondary exposure to other infected people. This in turn makes his or her system work in overtime mode to fight off the illness he or she is already suffering from. When children in turn come in contact with other carriers of disease, their health is compromised further, aggravating the original illness they may be carrying and must now fight off a new one.

What's ironic and all too common is that, as soon as you announce there will be a fun-filled day at the water park, your children's complaints of feeling ill mysteriously go away. Please take the time to reconsider your decision to allow them to join, especially if they have obvious signs of an illness or disease. Indicators to watch for include flu or cold-like symptoms, open sores, and discharge from natural openings, that is, ears, nose, throat, vaginal opening, urethra, and rectum. Also, the most common sign and symptom of all illness are nausea and vomiting.

Water parks and these illnesses is quite simply not a good match.

Stay home, get well, and then have fun.

Since I am having so much fun feeding on my own phobia, let's not stop. Let's say that after attending that attraction park, a day or two go by, and suddenly you or one of your family members begins to feel sick. Being the responsible parent you are, you take that loved one to the nearest medical facility. This could be your family doctor's office, outpatient clinic, or in the worst-case scenario, the emergency room. For the purpose of this scenario, which is played out every day, you soon find yourself shoulder-to-shoulder with strangers in a confined, confusing, and crowded waiting room, possibly for hours. Remember, this was preventable. There are only two reasons why others need to be in this patient-care setting: They are either sick, or they are treating the ill and injured. Reviewing what I mentioned earlier, it's the length of time and the proximity you are in to the infected host that determine the odds of you becoming a new host of that same disease.

There are other risk factors that are surrounding you. I am referring to the facility itself. The chair you're sitting in right now, reading this book, is contaminated with microorganisms. The arms and railings of the chair contain the highest concentration of microbes, more than other surfaces. The person that was occupying that chair prior to you may have been a carrier of an illness. I have never been in a medical facility where I witnessed someone from the janitorial staff immediately disinfecting these surfaces as soon as you got up. It's usually done after a complaint from a customer, or it's a timed procedure for the shift. So, indirect or cross-contamination is common in these types of environments.

Now you should ask yourself, what could possibly exist on these services I'm touching that are harboring a disease? I will answer that question for you. Most common are microbes from sneezing and coughing (Tuberculosis, Flu and Colds), mucous and sputum (Respiratory Diseases, Mono, Oral STD's), blood and other potentially infected fluids (Hepatitis, HIV), and open sores containing pus (MRSA, VISA)—all can exist on these hard surfaces.

I have observed in many situations women who put their purses down on the floor surface, just to pick it up later and place it in their laps or on the counter while they sign in. A more critical cargo is people. How many times have you witnessed parents allowing their children to crawl on the floor and then pick up a toy or book and put it directly in their mouth? The parent's response most likely was, "Honey, come here and give Mommy a big kiss; you'll be okay." *Get my point yet?*

I will now stop beating up on medical facilities, or maybe not. You see, we have left out probably the most daunting and persistent disease invading medical facilities all over the world today. This disease is advertised daily in medical journals, case studies, and the media, and it's not for the shock factor. MRSA, which stands for Methicillin-Resistant Staphylococcus Aureus or the "flesh-eating" disease, is perched in every medical facility ready to attack its next victim. Now that we are on the topic, let's discuss some serious issues the entire medical community and its patients are faced with. MRSA is a disease of opportunity. It can survive outside the living host for long periods of time, unlike some microorganisms that die off very quickly because of the undesirable environment in which it exists. Something as simple as a change in temperature, humidity, light (ultraviolet lighting), or even oxygen levels ($O2$) can eradicate or destroy this ominous bacterium. MRSA can hide on surfaces overlooked during routine cleaning operations. Unseen by the human eye, it may be present under furniture, windowsills, phones, keyboards, writing utensils, medical equipment, linen, latrines, and even clothing or jewelry. Now repeating what I said earlier, don't assume that even trained janitorial employees ("staff") are eliminating *staph*. Was that a pun?

We must take on the responsibility ourselves and be more observant of our surroundings and the hygienic practices of employees and the people that surround you. Medical facilities have some of the most stringent cleaning and decontamination standards of all industries. So why, in the United States of America, a Country of knowledge, wealth, and the most advanced medical facilities and practices in the world, still result in over 165,000 cases, that are medically acquired diseases by patients who didn't have that infection or infections prior to their stay? Of those cases confirmed, nearly 50 percent resulted in loss of limb, physical disability, or death, according to the CDC and the MMWR. The steps you need to take in preventing infection and becoming the next statistic will take patience and discipline. By following these easy but unorthodox procedures, you will decrease your chances of being exposed to these life-threatening diseases.

In situations where you have time before your medical visit, do your homework and get as much information as you can about the facility. All licensed clinics, hospitals, doctor offices, and dental facilities must adhere to strict State and Federal OSHA (Occupational Safety and Health Administration) reporting and documenting procedures for suspected cases of exposure incidents within that place of business. The primary online sites the general public has access to—www.cdc. gov, www.nih.gov, www.who.org, and www.cdc.gov/mmwr/—list and describe those guidelines. These sites can lead you to other sources and sidebar topics with related statistics.

Though information on positive test cases must remain anonymous, other related information must be documented, such as the number of cases confirmed, the medical facility reporting, and if possible, the means of transmission. All hospitals are ranked in a number of different categories, such as number of deaths, cases of transmittable diseases, pre- and post-op complications, lawsuits, status of licenses and certifications, OSHA investigations and findings, scope of practice, and overall comparative ranking. For example, hospital XYZ could be ranked #10 in the United States for the lowest number of mortalities.

Once you have found a reputable and safe facility, your next discipline is to observe your surroundings while asking yourself a few questions. What is the check-in procedure, and does it meet or exceed patient safety laws? Do they accommodate the patient with separate rooms, dividers, or open counters for signing in? Does the medical facility have waiting areas that are away from the general public but allow you to hear your name when called? Remember, it's the proximity and length of time you are exposed to these closed and potentially infectious areas that increase your chances for exposure.

When signing in, try using your own writing tool. I would bet that quite a few hands and mouths have been on the ones used by the medical staff. If by chance they provide disinfectant wipes, foams, or sprays, *use them*! If you happen to be carrying around your own, that's even better. The more times the same type of disinfectant is used, the greater the chance for disease-resistant strains to develop. Your product will be the new kid on the block. If you observe patients coughing or sneezing, the proper medical procedure for someone experiencing these symptoms with an undetermined cause is to isolate the patient from the general populace. However, that usually is impossible because of the lack of space. So ask the nursing staff for a face mask. Your nose and mouth will then be protected from any microscopic particles in the air that could end up in your lungs and your bloodstream.

Now that the paperwork is complete, typically you will find an open seat and grab something to read, such as a magazine, newspaper, or even a book. Put it down, unless you have just picked up a bible. Those surfaces are full of bacteria and other germs that can cause illness and aggravate any current medical issue you may be dealing with. Too many hands have been touching those materials. What I recommend to you is to bring your own reading source.

Now, time has gone by, and you suddenly realize you must use the lavatory. Why not just walk into the middle of a firefight in Afghanistan? Your chance of getting hit by a microbe bomb far exceeds your chances of being shot as a visitor in that country. I don't know about you, but I'm not a gambler nor do I play Russian roulette with my health or life. If you must relieve yourself, try to find a restroom as far away from the emergency room as you can. The road less traveled in this case is much safer.

Your name is finally called to be seen. Regardless whether the attending medical staff know you or not, consider this: when someone is having to deal with a high volume of patients or is bound to strict time frames, the first thing that's overlooked is good sound hygienic practices. You are no exception. When out of sight, out of mind. Since we don't have X-ray or MRI capabilities with our vision nor can we smell, feel, or taste these invaders, it's easy for janitorial staff to lower their guard and forego what is time consuming and costly. The formula is easy: more patients = more revenue = job security = more money.

Safety precautions that your health-care provider should be using include but are not limited to wearing gloves before physical contact and using disinfectants on all medical equipment before use to eliminate cross-contamination, with proper disposal of all medical supplies that have been used on a patient during medical procedures.

Allow me to share just one quick story of an obvious disregard for my safety that occurred recently during a visit to my dentist's office. After sitting down in the exam chair, I noticed the hygienist had already gloved up prior to entering the room. How many other potentially infected surfaces did she touch before placing her hands in my mouth? Also, the dental tools had already been opened and were just sitting on a surgical tray on top of a towel, completely exposed to the circulating air for what could have been a half hour or more. Every patient has the right to speak up and request to have the dental equipment in this case opened in front of you. During the procedure, the hygienist was handed a clipboard by another staff member and never removed her gloves to sign it.

Because of my personal cell count levels, my doctors have already said to me, "Rich, you're a bleeder." My coagulation capabilities are very low. Even a simple cleaning between my cheek and gums can cause severe bleeding. The dental hygienist just put others at risk of infection if I happened to have been a carrier of a disease at that time. I was initially the potential risk factor to the hygienist, being a bleeder, but by not removing her gloves when touching the clipboard, she puts me at risk of disease because of the open wounds in my mouth. These are just a couple examples that could have led to exposure and transmission of many different types of disease to me or others; such situations happen every day. Be more observant and don't be afraid to make requests. If they want to keep your business, they will listen to your demands.

School settings aren't any better. With thousands of kids entering and leaving campuses all over the United States nearly every day, it is inevitable that at some point a student will bring to school a disease that will pose a threat to anyone he or she has contact with. State Transit Authorities have reported that on any given day, there are 167,000 round-trip bus rides to and from all schools throughout the United States. These environments vary greatly with climate control. Some are cold and clammy and others hot and humid. All buses have closed circulatory systems that can harbor airborne and blood-borne diseases.

For years, parents have acquired a false sense of security, believing that the safety and well-being of their children are monitored correctly by teachers and school officials. Adding to this false sense of security are parents who are putting too much confidence in vaccinations, inoculations, and immunizations. Those preventative medical procedures only protect a person from the specific disease he or she was inoculated for. There are many other disease-causing microbes that could still infect your child.

Schools are a breeding ground for all disease, especially sexually transmittable diseases (STD). I will discuss that in greater detail in Chapter 4, "What Is Your Child Doing Behind the Racquetball Wall?" After considerable exhausting research, I set a goal to determine if, in fact, these diseases were being passed from one student to another at school. I needed to educate myself and others as to how many of these social diseases were jumping from one human host to another. Finally, I needed concrete proof of the number of victims infected during school activities. The first part of my investigation was to identify the source of transmission. Was the environment to blame for the existence of disease, or was it some specific type of physical contact one host had with another?

Although our children attend school to learn how to read and write, I found the housekeeping to be nothing to write home about. What I discovered first, to no surprise to me, was that the janitorial services and cleaning procedures fell well below cleaning guidelines with environmental and hygiene compliance laws. It's not a secret that large school districts rely on a bidding process (Request for Quote, RFQ) for these services under contract, which is often awarded to the lowest bidder. We all know the old saying "You get what you pay for." After conducting numerous visual inspections of these facilities—again, district and school names are withheld for disclaimer reasons—what I discovered was nothing short of "janitorial malpractice".

I would have felt safer going into the restrooms in a large metropolitan train depot than in some of these schools. It wasn't difficult to notice that certain parts of the floor were not mopped appropriately, if at all. This was especially noticeable around the toilets, washbasins, doorknobs, sink handles, and flushers. All of these surfaces need the most attention because they are touched the most by human hands. Many students I interviewed were just as concerned as I was for their safety. Many of the students used paper towels when touching these devices and even resorted to using their feet. That also is concerning to me because the bottom of your shoes carry all of those germs picked up from the floor, which are now hiding in the crevices and tread of your footwear. All these floor microbes would now be transferred to these restroom surfaces.

The classrooms weren't any better. If this next section taps into your phobia, you can skip it. We all have experienced this at least once in our lives, when a simple laugh or sneeze causes an uncontrollable relaxation of our bladder muscle or sphincter muscle (rectal). Those fluids or secretions now end up on the seat cover, which will eventually be used by another student in another class period. Speaking of periods, unfortunately when a female is going through her menstrual cycle, there may be a tendency to leave the tampon or pad in place for too long. The tampon or pad becomes oversaturated with menstrual fluids, contaminating the surfaces of the equipment. There is a reason why female products have warning labels on them. These warnings protect the consumer and ensure the products' proper use. Another reason for following the guidelines of your particular feminine product is that you will have protected yourself from complications like toxic shock syndrome (TSS), which is the poisoning of blood cells and can be fatal.

What I found under the desks was also startling—bubblegum

heaven. Remember, I stated that the mouth is the most infectious natural orifice of the human body, which is exactly where that gum came from. Other findings were other sticky candies, chew, and nasal secretions (boogers). For reasons unknown, the cleaning staff seemed to overlook these surfaces.

As I pondered my next journey through this disease-riddled battlefield, I suddenly heard loud noises and cheering coming from the gym. What could possibly pose a risk to my child in a gym other than a physical or emotional injury? After close examination of the sport courts, bleachers, locker rooms, showers, latrines, and water sources, such as pools and saunas, I was able to detect dozens of potentially infectious agents. Bacteria and viruses thrive in moist, humid environments. These microorganisms are in many cases extremely viable outside the human host. According to research conducted by the Wilderness Medical Society, they claim that in order to guarantee the complete destruction of all pathogens in water, the temperatures must excess 160 degrees. I don't know what your tolerance level is to hot water, but I personally can only handle temperatures of about 100 to 104 degrees. Again, we are at the mercy of the pool service, which should be using the appropriate amounts of chlorine and acid for the amount of water in that water source in order to kill these diseases upon contact.

If your child comes home one day with Herpes of the eyes or severe Pinkeye, you now have an idea where he or she may have gotten it. It was simply that last head dip underwater before they got out. Again, inquire as to the pool service the school currently contracts. You have the right to request to see the service dates and the chemical treatments they perform at each water source throughout the campus. For now, let's identify some of the more common diseases discovered in these settings that are reported routinely to the local Health Departments and the CDC: Pinkeye, Hepatitis, Herpes, and MRSA.

Last year I came across an article written by a researcher with the

CDC. The topic was Methicillin-Resistant Staphylococcus Aureas. This particular article spurred my interest in the ways in which athletes could be exposed and possibly infected with this flesh-eating disease. What first came to my mind was skin-to-skin contact. All athletes who participate in any form of contact sports could be at risk. So, how do we protect our athletes and other students who are exposed to these environments? They have to participate in physical education (PE) or play after-school sports. The first level of safety starts with the coaches and trainers. This is done through awareness and education.

When I am conducting infectious disease seminars, I am approached with several questions, including: What is MRSA? Are there different types? How is it transmitted? What are the symptoms? Let me answer some of those questions now.

MRSA, often called "staph" or "flesh-eating" disease, is a bacterium that is most commonly found in the nose or on the skin. The "resistant" simply refers to its ability to become immune to the antibiotics used to treat MRSA. In the case of MRSA, it is the antibiotic Methicillin. The other flesh-eating virus, called VISA, is resistant to a powerful antibiotic, Vancomycin. These skin infections may appear as sores or boils that often turn red, swollen, and painful or have pus and other drainage. Typically, MRSA occurs where there is a break in the skin, such as abrasions or minor cuts and burns, and areas of the body that have a lot of hair or where you itch frequently. These sites would include the back of your neck, wrists, ankles, and genitalia. MRSA skin infections typically can be treated with outpatient antibiotics, drainage of the pus pockets, and wound care. More serious cases can lead to systemic complications, such as pneumonia, bone infections, and eventually the breakdown of the dermis, sub-dermis, muscle tissue, and bone matter. Hence the term"flesh-eating."

The following sports appear to pose the greatest risks to athletes:

football, soccer, rugby, wrestling, field hockey, martial arts and fencing.

All athletes, regardless of the sport they participate in, should always practice good personal hygiene. This includes washing hands frequently with soap and warm water and applying an alcohol-based hand spray or foam. These hygiene techniques are particularly important after participating in sporting activities, after exchanging sports equipment, and after changing saturated wound-care products. Immediately take a shower after practice, and don't share soap or towels. Wash your uniform, clothes, and undergarments after each use. If you skip these steps, you're giving these microbes, in this case MRSA, the opportunity to thrive, reproduce, and spread to other surfaces.

In 2009, football athletes at Huntington Beach High School in Southern California reported an outbreak of MRSA, infecting over a dozen players, that was later linked back to the shoulder pads that were being shared and not cleaned according to the manufacturer's guidelines. Speak up and ask questions of the athletic directors and coaches. How are they protecting your child's safety and health?

CHAPTER 3
THE CHAIN OF TRANSMISSION

The most pressing global issue that comes to my mind is: What is happening in the vast arena of infectious diseases? Many experts speculate that we are gaining control in the fight against disease. Their justification is the advancements the medical communities worldwide have achieved and the scientific discoveries that have catapulted the United States to the forefront in the ever-changing atmosphere of this microbial world. Every day, every twenty minutes, we discover a new disease or the alter ego of existing pathogens somewhere around the globe. Are we really keeping up with the continual presence and onslaught of disease, or will we just be sitting ducks when the next pandemic occurs?

The first two chapters of this book have demonstrated that epidemics and pandemics from the past could resurface and have catastrophic effects on individuals and entire regions of the world. We have also provided education and awareness of the social microbe factories that surround us everywhere. Our daily routines predispose us to disease. You can protect yourself from these risk factors through awareness and resources we have discussed earlier. So now, as we move on to the core of this educational process, I am going to explain exactly how all infectious diseases are passed on from one human host to another.

This excludes diseases such as Heart Disease, Diabetes, Cancers, or any other conditions identified as a disease by the FDA, CDC, NIH, and WHO. I will be referring only to infectious disease that can lead to illness and death.

From a scientific standpoint, I'm expecting the world to undergo a catastrophic event we have never experienced before. But in the following chapters, I'm going to attempt to prove myself wrong. As you look around your environment, sometimes the threat is obvious. It could be an environment that has poor hygienic practices, such as public restrooms. It could be a surface, such as a bathroom door handle that has been touched by multiple customers.

All too often, media sources will report on a new drug that claims to be a cure against a specific disease or medical condition. Pharmaceutical companies also announce therapies that promise to get rid of the symptoms and illnesses that have invaded your body. With the blessing of the FDA, companies have introduced vitamins, drugs, compounds, potions, and many other substances that claim to relieve pain and eliminate and control symptoms, giving you the notion you're cured.

How many times have you read an article about some research that said, for instance, if you take this product as prescribed, it will prevent certain conditions from developing or prolong your good health? Then a few years later, a report is issued contradicting the original claim. This recently occurred with vitamin E, which claimed to slow down the development of prostate cancer. Then, after extensive case studies, researchers discovered it actually increased your chances of developing the same cancer. This was verified in The Journal of the American Medial Association (JAMA) in October 2011. After these new findings were reported, the manufacturers of this vitamin responded back to the public with the response that came across to me as, "*Whoops!* We made a mistake and apologize for any inconvenience this may have caused you. In the same breath, they didn't forget to thank you for the millions of dollars you infused into their bank accounts."

Industry-wide, however, there is a growing level of pessimism, whose voice is growing louder and more discouraging daily. It's not that we lack the resources and technology to make the necessary advancements to gain control with diseases. What is undermining our efforts is the political red tape, regulatory agencies, research and development companies, and the pharmaceutical industry.

For decades, we have slowly made strides in the mysterious world of microbes and have gained a basic understanding of their ability to coexist with the human race. The most pressing question is how all disease can be passed on from the environment to us and from one human host to another. Is it a typical behavior that allowed for transmission, a particular individual (with poor hygiene) that you had physical contact with, or maybe the environment or space you're occupying that caused you to intrude on their domain? Multiple watch groups have kept a close eye on the progress and the research currently being undertaken by pharmaceutical conglomerates, only to discover we are actually failing to develop new means to possibly eradicate these enemies.

What we know for sure is that there are certain elements that must be present and have to occur in order for any disease to be passed on from one human host to another. Is it simply a particular behavior that enables transmission of the disease? Maybe it's the type of person that you're being exposed to or coming in contact with. Do the elements of your surroundings have any influence on whether or not you're going to succumb to a particular disease?

The first link in the chain of transmission is that the person must be infectious at the time in which you're coming in contact with him. If he or she is not infectious as a carrier, regardless of the disease, that person cannot pass on the disease to you as a new host. The key element here is that the person is not just *infected* but is also *infectious*. There is a major difference between the two. Defining a person as "infected" means they have been exposed to a particular disease from another person or came in contact with it on a surface they touched and it now resides in their body. This individual is now a carrier of that disease and may not be aware of it. Once they have been infected, there will be a period of time in which symptoms won't be present. The disease is either in an incubation period (I refer to this as a hibernation period), or the virus or bacterium is in a dormancy state. In either case, that person is not capable of transmitting the disease to anyone else. When a person is "infectious," the virus or bacterium is active and reproducing in that persons body fluids and looking for its survival source. Typically that would be certain cells it can overtake and use as a microorganism factory. One of the first obstacles you are now faced with is to identify whether or not this person you are having casual or intimate contact with is infectious or noninfectious. If they are noninfectious, then a transfer of their disease is physically impossible.

Of course, in the scientific community, we have numerous ways to determine if a person is a health risk. We can take a blood test, urine, fecal samples, X-ray's, cat scans, ultrasounds, MRI's, or diagnose symptomatic changes in the body as an indicator of an illness or condition. Obviously, I don't always have access to these diagnostic tools, so I assume, regardless of whether or not he or she is experiencing an illness or exhibiting any signs or symptoms, they still have the potential to be infectious to me and others.

I never discriminate when it comes to disease. Regardless of your appearance, skin color, age, sex, political affiliation, or religious beliefs, you're still a risk to me. Approach everyone as a potentially infectious host. Use universal precautions.

Most experts agree that people are most infectious twenty-four hours before symptoms actually begin and up to forty-eight hours after symptoms cease. It's during these time frames when we are most susceptible to becoming infected ourselves. Common sense tells me that, when a person has a fever, nausea and vomiting, diarrhea, and other symptoms, I should avoid contact and exposure with him or her at all costs. Again, that's when we're most vulnerable.

The second link in the chain of transmission is that, regardless of what the body fluid or secretion is there still must be enough of the bacteria or virus present in those bodily secretions to be transmittable. How much is enough? Researchers and scientists have yet to decipher with years of testing under their belts and in their petri dishes, the viral or bacterial loading necessary for any disease to jump from one host to another. Is it just one particle, a hundred, a thousand, or a million?

There is a calibration formula we use in the research community to detect the amount of viral and bacterial loading in a fluid sample, which indicates the presence and volume of a microorganism. But again, what level or amounts of the disease is needed for a successful transmission? This mystery hasn't yet been solved. How important would those findings be to society as a whole? The reason why I sound somewhat callous is because universal precautions should be applied anytime you have exposure to any bodily fluid or secretion, regardless of the amount. But just for the sake of argument, let's put this research in motion.

In order to identify and publish this type of research, you would have to take an uninfected human being or animal (sorry, advocates for the humane treatment of animals) or a test tube sample and intentionally contaminate it with the disease being researched. Let's say hypothetically that recently a new strain of hepatitis was discovered and scientists were asked by the Centers for Disease Control and Prevention (CDC) or the World Health Organization (WHO) to independently determine for public awareness the life expectancy of the virus outside the human host. I reiterate throughout this book that what happens in a test tube or a laboratory setting isn't necessarily the same in the human body or other specimens as it relates to the existence of a living host. In order to determine the amount of viral loading in any particular body fluid that could lead to transmission, you would have to take a live sample of the disease and inject it into the bloodstream of someone who's not infected and see if it takes.

For our first test, let's say we isolated just one particle of the Hepatitis B Virus. After introducing it into the host's bloodstream, the researchers would wait for the appropriate time before testing the serum in the new host. When the results came back negative, we would record, it didn't take. So for our next attempt, we would inject one thousand particles of the virus, and again it might fail. The third effort would utilize 1 million particles, and still we could get negative results. Understand that scientists and researchers almost never concede defeat. So we would keep increasing the viral loading to a level that would finally result in a positive test. Who would volunteer for that type of research? *Nobody!*

So, is one particle enough? We will probably never know the answer to these questions. For decades, we have relied on scientific research involving many different species of animals. This doesn't necessarily coincide with human research.

The third link in the chain of transmission is that there must be a portal of entry by which this disease, whether it's a virus or bacteria, can get into your body. What exactly is the definition of a "portal of entry"? A portal of entry is simply any open avenue into your system that these microbes can utilize. As you remember, I said that your skin was your first and most effective barrier in your fight against disease. Well, if the continuity of the skin is disrupted in any way, then you are at risk. This could involve a burn that has penetrated the top layer of the skin. Maybe you have blisters from a sunburn that have broken open. That's a portal of entry. I'm sure many of you go out and you get manicures and pedicures. Every time you do so, they open up microscopic wounds between the cuticles and the nail beds themselves. If you were to come in contact with someone's bodily secretions to those areas, could it be a large enough opening for that disease to enter? *Yes!* Remember, we are discussing microscopic organisms.

How many of you floss your teeth on a regular or semi regular basis? I would hope all of you. Every time you floss your teeth, you're opening up microscopic wounds between the gum lines and the teeth themselves. So if you were to get, again, someone's body fluids in your mouth, even through casual kissing, you could be at risk. That could be a large enough opening for these tiny little microscopic organisms to get into your system.

Another avenue by which infectious diseases may enter is through cuts, tears, lesions, evulsions, eviscerations, or any other breakdown in the continuity of the skin, including microscopic openings.

You should always inspect your own body surface, constantly looking for possibly injuries or openings that may become the freeway into your system. When you are in the stages of undress, take the time to look over the areas I discussed earlier. Think of it as preventive medicine.

A more common way for these microbes and microorganisms to get into your body is through natural orifices. These natural openings would include your eyes, ears, nose, mouth, vaginal opening, rectum, and even the tip of the penis, meaning the urethra. These openings are what I call "the Panama Canals of disease."

The research that I was involved with years ago startled me with the fact that these openings can be microscopic in size as well. To give you a simple example of the size of these microorganisms, you could take just a teaspoon of blood, and with a micron/electron microscope, isolate approximately one billion particles of hepatitis in just one teaspoon. So, how big of an opening must exist? It could be as small as a pinhole. You may not even realize that you have been exposed this way because you can't feel it. It's not actively bleeding, and you're not even aware of the opening yourself. These openings can exist inside your natural orifices.

The fourth and final link in the chain of transmission is that there has to be some way in which that microorganism can gain access to your bloodstream. That's why we term these "blood-borne pathogens." That's where they must finally reside. This is where the reproduction process occurs. I refer to your blood serum as a disease factory; from there, microorganisms can spread to other body fluids or organs within your body. These body fluids could include vaginal secretions, semen, breast milk, nasal secretions, vomit, fecal matter, urine, cerebral spinal fluids, peritoneal, synovial fluids, and even bone marrow. In fact, that is where your blood cells develop. Once the pathogen becomes active, you are now infectious to others, typically within twenty-four hours after exposure. Keep in mind that if this were related to an airborne pathogen, it's just simply through the efforts of breathing that it can enter your bloodstream through the mucous membrane linings in your nose and, of course, the back of your throat, which leads directly to your bloodstream.

So to put this entire chain of transmission into perspective, let's create a real-life scenario we all have experienced. *Step 1*: You're meeting a business associate or personal friend for lunch. At the time of this visit, your friend appears to have a mild cough. So you politely ask if she is feeling okay, and she responds back that she's fine, it's nothing to worry about. You've just come in contact with a particular individual who at that time is potentially infectious. In other words, that disease she's carrying in her body is active and transmittable through coughing. The diseases will simply piggy back on her respiratory molecules, which you now breathe into your lungs. Hopefully it's just a cold or flu and not something more serious like tuberculosis (TB). *Step 2*: There's enough of the disease in the body fluid or secretion that you've now came in contact with to be transmittable. *Step 3*: There is a portal of entry into your body, meaning there is a natural opening or a breakdown in the continuity of your skin. *Step 4*: Somehow that microorganism gained access into your bloodstream. The chain of transmission is now complete. Congratulations, you are now a new host of her disease.

Assuming this happened to you, would you know right away that you were just infected with a medical condition or disease from that person? Most of the time, it would be virtually impossible to determine what person or surface point infected you. Would you wake up the next morning with this sudden burden of weight to your side? Or immediately have this sharp pain to your shoulder? No, it takes time for any symptoms to begin, unless it's food poisoning.

Suppose that in a unique situation, both of you go to your respective doctors' offices, explain what just occurred, and the doctor would recommend a particular test to see what transpired. Remember, however, that you're testing way too soon after the exposure incident. Even if the test results were negative, it could be a false negative because you were testing in the earliest stages of the disease's life. There typically wouldn't be enough viral or bacterial loading to be detectable. You might have to wait weeks or months and follow up with a confirmatory test. This test would simply confirm the first results as being true negative or true positive. If one of you had tested positive on the original screening, you were already a carrier and got the disease somewhere else and from another host.

As I've mentioned throughout this book, your goal is to somehow identify and thereby eliminate just one of those elements in the chain of transmission. If you can break just one of these vital links, a transmission is physically impossible. You will never be infected. So it is conceivable that a person could actually lead a disease-free life. There is a controversy in the scientific world where those who believe that staying well and never being sick could predispose us to the catastrophic effects of a future illness that our immune system would not be capable of responding to. The other side of this theory is that one can create an impenetrable immune system that has an arsenal of immune helper cells to prevent any disease from invading, stabilizing, and destroying its host, *you*. Social microbial factories and sexual behavior are not the only culprits that can pass on disease.

The history of epidemiology has demonstrated numerous times that most plagues, epidemics, and pandemics were the direct result of the mating of two different diseases or a change in a single microbe's genetic makeup (mutation). War events from our past, such as World War I, World War II, Vietnam, the Gulf War Desert Shield/Storm, and the Iraqi War, have proven that when a major conflict arises, the movements of our ground forces spreads infection quickly around the war zone. The concentration of troops, military officials, and civilians coexisting with movements in and out of the fighting arena can spread diseases to other communities, cities, and countries, sometimes the same day.

Many pathogens existed only in isolated, small regions of the world for years. The United States and other United Nations members sent scientists to these regions months prior to the troops' arrival. Their mission was complex. The critical element was to determine through sample studies, hospital reports, and genetic mapping the presence of any disease we had not yet discovered or new strains and mutations of existing pathogens that we could develop vaccines for to protect any personnel entering the region. Suddenly preventive medicine was going to be used on a scale never attempted before and would be mandatory, not voluntary. Unlike the flu shots made available every year to anyone choosing to take them, the vaccines had to be streamlined and put on the fast track for approval by the FDA. This practice of expediting vaccines is not common practice, but it was time sensitive because of the presidential order to occupy this region to eliminate terrorist cells at the time.

This information immediately put up a warning signal to me that a disease existing in a region of the world not heavily traveled by the West could go unidentified. The rotation of troops, civilians, and officials leaving that region to return to their homes, may have picked up a pathogen in a carry-on bag which now just became a first-class ticket to any destination in the world. For a mere carry on fee, anyone could transport a life-threatening microbe back to his or her families, only to then be transmitted to friends and colleagues.

This scenario, I hope, gives you a greater sense of urgency and responsibility to be more observant of the people and surroundings that potentially could become a health risk to you. Again, don't become that first documented case. The chain of transmission is sensitive to the four elements I listed for you in this chapter. If just one of those links is disrupted, you are not at risk. We unfortunately put ourselves in harm's way every day without realizing it. Before we leave this chapter and move on to the steps that will give you the knowledge, skills, and resources to break the chain of disease, I want you to participate in a small test. Don't worry, I'm not going to have you fill anything out and mail it in to me for grading. If you're like my wife, who gets extremely nervous before tests—and her grades usually were reflective of this disposition—you can evaluate yourself.

What I am asking you to do is simple, and you can pick or choose the task you feel most comfortable with. Here are your tasks:

- Take the loose change or bills out of your purse and place them in your mouth.
- Go to your bathroom and lick the doorknob.
- Place a piece of the outer skin of a fruit or vegetable without washing it in your mouth.
- Put your hand on the phone, keyboard, or writing utensil from your office, and then wipe your eyes.
- Remove your shoes from the bottom with your bare hands, and then go back to the snack you were eating and finish it.

How are we doing so far? Do you feel comfortable and safe? Since it's your home and your personal items, you most likely think you're not at risk of disease. After all, you've been told by many of your friends and relatives that your home is so tidy and clean.

Next time you're at the grocery store, eating in a restaurant, sitting in the waiting area of the emergency room with your child, or shaking a stranger's hand, remember this exercise. No environment or surface is 100 percent disease-free. Only sterile environments can make that disclaimer.

Now, in order for you to have aced the test, you shouldn't have done any of those tasks. The scary thing is that you do these things every day without realizing it. Touching contaminated surfaces and then scratching your eyes or putting your fingers in your mouth are all too common places. Already you could have exercised hygienic practices that keep those links in the chain of transmission intact.

Please take the time to be more observant of the people and surroundings you eventually have contact with and put into action the steps that can prevent you from being in harm's way. Get disciplined and change these high-risk habits. Like anything else in life, it takes knowledge, sound thinking, and action.

CHAPTER 4
WHAT IS YOUR CHILD DOING
BEHIND THE RACQUETBALL WALL?

The chapter's title says it all. If you are a concerned parent and curious about the level of participation in sexuality or other promiscuous acts your child is doing away from home, you need to sit down. The following is not designed with the scared straight approach to this pressing issue. It's simply to shed light on the behavioral changes that have occurred the last few years with teens and young adults.

Even the most prominent researchers, psychologists, behavioral scientists, and counselors have been thrown a curveball. Why has the sexual behavior of this generation's adolescents changed so drastically? As I investigated these changes and patterns of sexual behavior among teens, I determined there were two common denominators shared by all who participate in the sexual activity we will address in this chapter.

The First Common Denominator: Age has little or no influence on the level of sexual activity children choose to engage with.

The Second Common Denominator: Due to the lack of education and knowledge, there appears to be a sheer disregard of the consequences they face. Street smarts will not protect you in these situations. Sexually transmitted diseases don't recognize how old you are, what your skin color is, whether you're male or female, or what your sexual preference is.

The behavior I will describe in this chapter will startle you. It should be every parent's concern, not nightmare, to realize this could be your child we are comparing notes about. It reminds me of the good old days when you couldn't wait to open the letter on your desk before class or taped to your sports locker before practice, sent to you by an admirer. I wish it were that innocent today. The techniques and tools our children utilize are far more sophisticated and stealth. How do we as educators, mentors, and most importantly parents supervise our children and others they associate with to monitor the behavior they engage in to keep them safe and healthy. The schools that are paid to educate our children to the guardians who raise them are losing control of the decision-making process of the youth of this generation. When I am lecturing on this subject, the response from attendees usually is mixed. Some are startled by the information, while others choose not to believe it. What I remind my audience of constantly is that my goal is not to change your beliefs, thought patterns, or political affiliations, nor is the information based on assumptions, speculations, or theories. The information is based on facts backed by case studies, research, and statistical information.

I have always believed the educational process should begin at home. But at what age should you consider sitting your children down for the "big talk"? This depends on a number of factors. First, do you feel comfortable taking on the responsibility of talking to your child about sex? Second, do you feel your child is mature enough to understand your message to practice either abstinence or *safer sex* approaches, whichever you believe to be the best for your child? Lastly, are your children willing to be upfront and honest about their sexuality? Some specialists believe that if you attempt to educate teens when they are too young, you may end up putting thoughts in their heads that were not there to begin with, thereby promoting certain sexual behavior prematurely.

The conversation my parents had with me occurred at age twelve. I was not sexually active yet and didn't quite understand the information or message they were conveying to me. I remember thinking that maybe there was something wrong with me because I hadn't even kissed a girl yet. So to hear about intercourse, oral copulation, french kissing, and how to excite a woman in different ways was overwhelming. That's when Hugh Hefner and I began a lifelong friendship. It's amazing how many life interests we shared. The pinup centerfolds became my avenue to the safest sex I could enjoy at that age. It cannot, however, be argued that the "birds and the bees" conversation has helped educate generations of people.

Human beings by nature have the desire, will, and need to feel happy. The desire to feel attractive to others brings along with it impulses not experienced every day. These feelings will eventually propel into actions that bring excitement, but also a degree of danger as well. To help you better understand these dangers, you need to inquire as to the sexual conduct your child is pursuing.

This may not be easy to accomplish. What I have found is that the youth of today have changed their means of communication and whom they communicate with, and have altered their content and language for social reasons and to remain anonymous.

The barriers you may encounter trying to dissect this vital information are many. The social network plays the greatest role in seducing our children to engage in sexual behavior never seen with other generations. They have access to cell phones, text messaging, social sites such as Facebook and Twitter, blogs, message boards (iVillage), and cliques or gangs that throw signs and have colors specific to their culture.

What doesn't surprise me is that mainstream media has also jumped on the bandwagon. Sex sells, and there is plenty for the taking. The competition is so intense that these companies go to the extreme to always stay on the cutting edge. Your child may be a victim of these marketing techniques and schemes, which have led to unwanted pregnancies, increased drug use, sexual promiscuity, and infection rates (STD's) that are at an all-time high.

The TV shows that air on major network stations that claim to help us understand and cope with the issues parents and educators are faced with daily only appear to exacerbate the problems. They too often glamorize the misfortunes, poor decisions, and tragic outcomes our youth experience due to their indiscreet actions.

According to the Centers for Disease Control and Prevention (CDC), under there Data and Statistic Report, approximately 4 million teens contract one or more STDs annually. The most prevalent are Herpes, Gonorrhea, Syphilis, and Chlamydia. Not far behind are Hepatitis and HIV.

Science Daily (www.Sciencedaily.com) has published the results of a survey that was designed to get a better understanding of the concerns teens have of acquiring STDs. What the research unveiled was that 92 percent interviewed indicated their greatest fear was being infected with STDs, which included HIV/AIDS. The scientific study did not limit its research to the types of STDs I have already mentioned. Other types indicated were Bacterial Vaginosis (BV) and Human Papillomavirus (HPV).

Unfortunately, the number of STD's continue to grow every year. The survey also identified that 51 percent of boys under the age of eighteen said they never used condoms during intercourse, with 47 percent of females not requiring their sexual partner to use a protective barrier during sex. Sexual intercourse is referring to vaginal, rectal, and oral penetration. Fifty percent of female teens don't use any form of birth control. The research that disturbed me the most was that 6 percent of girls and 8 percent of males had engaged in various forms of sexual intercourse before the age of fourteen. Again, what's your child doing behind the racquetball wall?

The Pacific Institute of Research and Evaluation took a more aggressive approach to the line of questioning about sexuality. It asked teens between the ages of twelve to sixteen to indicate the kind of sexual activity they have engaged in and estimated number of encounters. What was uncovered is that 80 percent performed acts of genital touching and believed they were still virgins, 70 percent said they retained their virginity after having oral sex, and 14 percent said that after having anal or vaginal sex they also saw themselves as virgins.

The gross misconception is that if they don't ejaculate inside the partner or have rectal penetration, she can't get pregnant, they are immune to disease, and they still are saving themselves for the right person. Rectal intercourse is one way to preserve their virginity but does not protect them from infectious diseases. Unfortunately this type of behavioral pattern is difficult to identify do to the lack of individuals willing to participate in these surveys. Since proper sex education is not being conducted in our schools or in our homes, children are left with peer pressure, intuition, or the "take-a-chance" approach that can result in high risk contact that can lead to transmission of infectious diseases.

I had an opportunity to sit in on a sex education course at my daughter's middle school when she was in the sixth grade. The teacher was to follow two pieces of paper that had been scripted by the school district's educational advisory board with the approval of the school board members, supervised by the PTA members.

What I listened to bordered on educational malpractice. The information was not only inaccurate and outdated but was misleading as well. It simply did not address the behavioral consequences the students could be faced with due to certain sexual acts. The diseases they would be most at risk of acquiring and how they could spread their disease to others were never discussed. When it came to the question and answer portion of the course, it was evident that the teacher hadn't received any formal training necessary to address the students' questions.

When I approached the school board members at an open meeting for the public to raise my concerns regarding the content of the course, I was immediately diverted to the State Officials who oversee the development of these courses. I also experienced a lot of resistance from PTA members and parents. They argued that this type of education should begin in the home and be reinforced by qualified, credentialed teachers. Great point, but this is not being done to the level the students need. Again, *ignorance is not bliss*; what your child doesn't know will eventually harm him or her.

Don't blame yourself for these unfortunate events. When I was approaching that vulnerable age, my parents had a difficult time deciding how they should pursue the educational process with my siblings and me about sex. Parents are immediately faced with the greatest obstacle of all, a deaf ear. The youth of today are more interested in and trust the word on the street than what is more formal, practical, and safe. Social pressure existed with past generations, but promiscuity has changed tremendously compared to the "Leave it to Beaver" era. The alarming rise in the number of cases of sexually transmitted diseases has statisticians scratching their heads as to the root cause. I feel comfortable blaming their friends for any unsafe sexual practices that cause youth harm.

After the conclusion of my research and that of many other reputable medical professionals, we gained a new perspective of the power these social groups, cliques, gangs, and youth sex clubs have on our children. It's obvious that gender, sex, age, social status, and safe sex practices don't make us immune to pathogens. There isn't any paradigm such as *safe sex*. If you are sexually active, you are always at risk of disease. *Safer sex* means just that. Simply using protection in all situations will decrease you and your partner's chances of infection. However, modifying your pattern of sexuality will decrease your level of safety simply because you have now strayed away from your normal routine, which gives you a false sense of security.

What I constantly hear during my consulting seminars from attendees is, "Richard, I have been doing the same thing with my partner or partners for years, and I have never had an STD!" That could be true, or perhaps you simply haven't yet developed symptoms, which could take years to surface. If you test routinely because of past behavior that made you suspicious of your own status, those results may also indicate a false negative result. During this incubation period, you could still pass on the disease that is in your system. Remember what I asked earlier in the book: "Have you ever been sick a day in your life and didn't know where you got it?"

As we mature, understanding and concern for the consequences we may be faced with change. Remember, the youth of today are beginning to experiment with their feelings and sexuality. For those of you who haven't kept up with the times, let's now take an eye-opening, jaw-dropping journey into the daily lives of our youth and the rewards or consequences they can earn by participating in promiscuous behavior.

Recently, I watched and listened to the author of a newly released book called "Oral Sex in the New Midnight Kiss" by Sharlene Azam. In her book she was identifying the sexual behavior of teens in Canada that came from affluent families, not the homeless or drug addicted. They were being recruited by there girlfriends to service up to as many as seven men a night, several times a week with sexual favors. The parents and their siblings had no clue that their daughter or sister was involved with this type of promiscuous behavior. This is not only isolated to the country of Canada. It is happening in the United States and many other countries around the world.

When I was going through my teens and early adolescent years, I had the notion that I was a mature male and was ready for sex. Little did I know that other factors undermined my plan. The partner with whom you share your first intimate moments too often causes you to try a sexual act you have never experienced that may put you at risk of disease. Maybe that first encounter was intimidating, or your partner was more experienced sexually, which led you to engage in a sexual act of their preference. So what's a hormonally imbalanced teenager to do but rely on friends? That's a mistake! You see, their preferences in a partner may be different than yours. After multiple encounters, slowly but surely, social pressure gains a firm grip on you, and ultimately your choices are someone else's. This leads me into the next chapter, which defines exactly what promiscuity means.

CHAPTER 5
SEXUAL PROMISCUITY GONE WILD

The root cause of the decisions our teens and adolescents are making today is do to social pressure. It takes "keeping up with the Jones's" to a whole different level. In order to remain a member of these social groups, you must play by their rules and that involve sexual promiscuity.

These groups are referred to as cliques, sex groups, gangs, and bands of teens that are identified with special monikers. These monikers have many different names, such as Bambies, Tool Girls, Wannabes, Train Riders, Over-Under Girls, Slutsational, Fluffers, and two more names too offensive and vulgar to keep this book rated PG. Each of these groups has a reputation for a certain type of initiation that allows others to be a member. The first is called "the lineup". The term gives away the act right away. After school or during a party, the girl who chooses to be part of this group will give oral copulation to as many boys as the leaders can line up for her. Oral sex is viewed so casually that it's the same as kissing. When the act is done, the new girl is now accepted into the group.

The problem with this behavior is obvious. The male participants often don't wear condoms because it's not cool, it's difficult to keep an erection in a non intimate setting, and they don't think they are at risk. It would be too easy to argue this behavior was performed out of complete ignorance. I should mention that it's always the person being penetrated that's at greatest risk of disease. In this case, the route into the girl's system could be sores in the mouth, like gingivitis, open wounds around the teeth and gums due to irregular or aggressive flossing, and dryness of the oral cavity and tongue. The male doesn't have to ejaculate in his partner's mouth to put her at risk. The presence of pre-cum, which is very common prior to orgasm, also can carry disease-causing microbes.

This again demonstrates the lack of education, ignorance, and the complete disregard for protecting yourself and your partner from disease. Nearly every day I receive e-mails and text messages through which I acquire information as to the latest trends occurring with our teens and adolescents. One of the hot topics in the media has been the alarming climb in teen pregnancies. The youth of today, realizing that they are not immune to this, have come up with some creative ways to avoid the risk of pregnancy yet still be sexually active. This behavior also protects their status as virgins. I am referring to rectal intercourse. Really? Ouch!

When both people involved have thoroughly discussed having rectal penetration, feel comfortable with their decision, and the timing and mood are just right, this could turn out to be a painful compromise. The rectum's primary function is to work as an exit route for anything that enters your body during consumption that your system doesn't need any longer. Let the truth be told, however: since there is no route from your rectum to the uterus, pregnancy is physically impossible. However, rectal intercourse is considered the second-highest risk in acquiring a sexually transmitted disease. Only vaginal penetration poses a greater risk. The problem with rectal intercourse is that the lining of the rectal wall is very fragile, and it is therefore susceptible to minor cuts, tears, and lesions caused by the friction of the penis during penetration. If ejaculation occurs without a condom, the person being penetrated is at risk of any disease that may be carried in the semen of the male partner. Now it has direct access to the female's bloodstream.

Let's talk a less-invasive act of sex. Hand jobs are often used to gratify a partner, just like masturbation. Since no penetration occurs with either partner, the participants again assume there is no risk involved. Wrong again! If one believes that one can take an unprotected hand to the male or female genitalia (skin-to-skin contact) and not be at risk, he or she is fooling him or herself. This type of sexual conduct occurs more frequently than you would imagine. These actions, which often are performed at school, usually occur under desks, in small sections of the grounds with students surrounding them as a guard, behind classrooms, in pool areas or locker rooms, and in cars in the parking lot. Skin-to-skin contact can lead to surface infections, cross-contamination, and finally if ejaculation is achieved, exposure to semen (men) and vaginal secretions (female) to your hand, other skin surfaces, or natural orifices such as eyes and mouth. Foreplay can be a hideaway for microscopic organisms which can harbor under your fingernail, jewelry, or the surface of your skin. These microbes are capable of attacking anything they come in contact with. The only advice I can give you is to use protection and wash your hands immediately with soap and hot water.

If I have been successful in spurring your curiosity and you're still with me, you're probably wondering if there are any signs that would indicate that young adults continue to engage in this behavior. Absolutely, but I'm not quite there yet. The most disturbing sexual behavior I have yet to fully understand was reported first by Law Officials in the state of Texas. Earlier in this chapter, I mentioned there were different groups of youth, each having its own moniker. The reports filed by the Gang Unit Detectives in Fort Worth, Texas, received verifiable information implicating two female Latino gangs of having unprotected sex with HIV-positive males to be accepted into the gang.

The initiation process was simple. It drew absolutely no attention from law enforcement, didn't involve innocent bystanders—which is often the case with drive-by shootings—and was witnessed only by their own gang members. The gang felt that the greatest demonstration of a person's need or willingness to be accepted into their sisterhood, "no pun intended", was to put her life at risk by having sex with a guy that had tested (confirmed) positive for the virus HIV. The act was witnessed by other gang members, and the initiate had to engage in three acts of sexual contact: oral copulation, rectal intercourse, and vaginal penetration.

What is most disturbing to me is that the perpetrator never uses protection and he must ejaculate in each natural orifice. The prospective gang banger would then wait approximately one month or until she could get into a free anonymous health clinic to be tested. If her results came back negative for HIV infection, she was in the gang. The problem with testing that quickly after contact is that she may still be in the incubation period. This is known as a false negative test result. That person will need to take a confirmatory test to prove the first test was accurate. If her result had returned positive for the HIV virus, she could still get into the gang by either killing a rival gang member or having unprotected sex with a rival gang member's boyfriend. Wow! Just when you thought you'd heard it all. This particular initiation has trickled into other Metropolitan areas, such as New York and Los Angeles.

This information definitely raises some questions for me as an educator. Could it be possible that more children have been seduced or misguided by social pressure, resulting in their participation with similar sexual behavior? Doctors with specialties in the field of Child Psychology have published findings based on case studies from their clients that validate this admitted behavior among our teens and adolescents. The purpose of identifying and sharing this factual information is to encourage parents to have an open dialogue with their children.

The following are indicators of certain sexual activities. For instance, color of wristband, shoes and shoe laces, nail polish and makeup colors tell others what they have done or are sexually into. This will allow other people to immediately identify someone who are willing and able to perform certain sexual acts.

Here are a few tips of the dress code changes you can look for with your own child. With clothing, he or she must be careful of color choices so as not to send a false signal or a gang affiliation and at the same time, stay in accordance with the school's own dress code rules. Children will make subtle changes to their wardrobe, such as flying their colors with wrist scarves or certain colored wrist bands. Those cancer survivor bands, soul-mate or charity wrist guards just took on a completely different meaning. I experienced this when volunteering for an American Heart Association walk or jog - athon to raise funds for heart disease and stroke awareness. It was quite obvious that the students that chose the red wrist band where identifying themselves to others, their level of sexual experience while the students who chose the green wrist bands where being classified as inexperienced but willing to experiment to avoid being shut out by the various groups. My knowledge of this comes from many years working with juvenal offenders and their probation officers who enlightened me as to the significance in the choice of colored wrist bands.

Shoes also come into play—by either tying the laces or leaving them open. Open shoes, of course, mean easy removal, quick action, and actively participating in sex. Remember the old saying "just another notch in my belt"? Decades later it still shares a similar meaning. The number of notches visible indicates how far or how many "bases" they are willing to go. The fourth notch or "base" is not all the way— that's still third base; fourth means multiple partners. Hairstyles may include braids or side and rear ponytails that are shifted to the other side after having sex, just like moving the tassel after graduation.

Nail polish colors and designs indicate different acts of sex. Sometimes girls will even give their partner a code or call name, much like a hunter calling out for his prey, and paint it on one or all of their nails. This leads me back to shoes. Typically girls wear open-toe shoes or sandals (flip-flops) to show off their color and signs. Lipstick colors and sheen gloss provide the potential partner a clear history of her sexuality. The higher gloss products are meant to resemble sexual fluids, and the color application shows her level of experience.

Is this as confusing to you as it is for me? Let's try this scenario. Let's say you are a student walking across the quad area over to the lunch section and you see a tenth grader wearing a green wristband with her shoes untied and pink fingernail polish with the ring finger containing the letters and number bj4. Her hair braid is on the left side of her head. She is missing an earring on that same side, and the thumb on her right hand contains six thin rings. All these signs indicate her past and present sexual preferences. Confusing, I know, but not to our youth. That's how they keep their sexual behavior stealth.

So far, we have uncovered a lot of the sexual behavior the young adults of today engage in and how they communicate their willingness to perform certain sexual favors. We also took a disturbing journey behind the racquetball wall and discovered the means by which they keep this behavior stealth or "under the covers." There is unfortunately one more issue we have yet to address that can lead a person into making destructive decisions that become an opportunity for disease to be passed on from one host to another, is the influence of alcohol and drugs. These two elements play a major role in the chain of transmission.

According to SADD (Students Against Destructive Decision) at www.sadd.com, alcohol and drug use have the greatest control and impact on our teens' decision-making process. Statistics show that sixth graders say their number one reason for having sex and using drugs is to rebel. Alcohol quickly affects the chemicals in the portion of their brains that controls emotions, inhibitions, and desire. SADD statistics show that drinking alcohol and drug use increases significantly between sixth and seventh grades. The influence of alcohol and the effect it has on the central nervous system (CNS) makes it easier for a person to make decisions he or she normally would avoid that could put him or her at risk of disease. Sexually transmitted diseases are just waiting for that opportune time to take the path of least resistance from their current host to the next via wet kissing, vaginal secretions (intercourse), and semen (oral).

As adolescents become older, the number of high-risk sex acts increases as some begin to experiment with alcohol and drugs. The amount of alcohol consumed may also rise, leading to impaired judgment, attention deficit disorders, numbing of sensory motor skills, and a decrease in rational thinking. Because alcohol is considered a depressive drug, a pick-me-up may be in order. Statistics show that drug use continues to rise during eighth and ninth grades. Drugs will then counteract the effects of alcohol and give a person more energy to pursue acts of affection and make it last longer. There are literally hundreds of street drugs, with many different slang names associated with them. However, the most popular category is stimulants, which range from legal energy boost drinks (caffeine) to narcotics, such as meth or cocaine.

As these habits of consumption of alcohol and drugs increase, SADD statistics indicate that sexual activity has resulted in a significant increase in STD cases among teens, adolescents and adults. Research also indicates that STDs are at their highest levels in decades. Some would argue that this increase is a result of the growth in population, not changes with promiscuity. Any person identified as having a sexually transmitted disease, including but not limited to Hepatitis, Herpes, and HIV/AIDS, must be reported to the health department and is public record. The identity of the person being reported is kept confidential except in the situation where a crime has been committed and the victim gives authorities permission to release his or her name publicly.

SADD has also compiled research that indicates sexual activity peaks in the eleventh and twelfth grades. These young adults are now extremely vulnerable to strangers who may take advantage of them because of their willingness to drink, use drugs, and participate in a sex act.

There has been an increase in sedatives called Roofies being used on unsuspecting, innocent victims. FYI, for those of you who are not familiar with this term, Roofies (Rohypnol) is Benzodiazapam, like the tranquilizer Valium. The drug can be dropped into any drink without notice. These popular date rape drugs produce a profound, prolonged sedation and short-term memory loss, which can last from eight to twenty-four hours. The reason why it's considered the drug of choice is its cost. The street value is between one to five dollars each. Other names from this category of drugs are Gamma Hydroxybutyric acid, (GHB), Gamma Butyrolactone, (GBL), Ketamine, Burundanga, and Scopolamine.

My advice to avoid intentional poisoning with these date rape drugs is:

- Never leave beverages unattended.
- Don't accept drinks from strangers.
- Only accept drinks from the bartender.
- Friends should look after friends.
- If someone appears drunk after consuming a small amount of alcohol, get him or her to a safe place.

Remember that intoxication is a major contributor of destructive decisions. Add to that a date rape drug, and you have the perfect recipe for disease exposure.

If you or someone else you know assumes they have been a victim of a date rape crime, that person should seek medical attention immediately. Never remove clothing, take a shower or douche prior to arriving at the medical facility. Medical staff will most likely want to test your urine and blood, do a vaginal culture swab, and give you a pregnancy test. Finally, the attending physician will ask you to submit to STD testing. I know this sounds intrusive, but it is necessary, so they can provide you with the appropriate treatment and retain baseline test results for comparison with any follow-up testing.

As we identified in this chapter, you can take the appropriate steps to prevent exposure to a potentially infectious individual by altering the way you interact and modifying your lifestyle. You can make sound, responsible decisions by avoiding high-risk behavior that can lead you to a risky, harmful, and potentially life-threatening situation. Finally, avoid alcohol and drugs, which can also alter your ability to make safe choices. Don't become the next statistic!

CHAPTER 6
PROTECTIVE EQUIPMENT
AND PERSONAL HYGIENE

The most efficient and cost-efficient way you can decrease or eliminate your chances of coming in contact with a potentially infectious person and also prevent any contact with his or her disease-carrying bodily fluids or secretions is barriers. You also can take the route of abstinence. This is a choice everyone can make. For those of you who will take the lower road and choose to be sexually active, I'm going to provide you with constructive alternatives that will replace high-risk, promiscuous behavior with techniques that will allow you to stay sexually active and feel sexually attractive while offering protection from disease. Obviously I believe the use of personal protective products and aggressive personal hygiene practices is the most critical factor one can utilize to increase his or her level of safety. Regardless of your activity, whether it is professional or socially related, personal protective equipment is essential in breaking the chain of transmission.

Regarding socially transmitted diseases, there are two ways in which one could protect him or herself, the first being common sense. Common sense, of course, is derived through direct education of the risk factors you may be faced with at the time of exposure. The second way you can protect yourself is by implementing the use of protective barriers.

What I have done is categorize sexual behavior or acts of affection into four categories, starting with no-risk activities and leading up to high-risk activities.

It is important for you and your partner to understand which activities can increase your chances of getting certain STDs.

No Risk:

- Hugging
- Masturbating alone
- Dry kissing

Low Risk:

- French or wet kissing: This is generally safe if there are no open sores or cuts on the lips or mouth. Wet kissing and licking of the entire body can be sexually arousing. Just remember to avoid natural orifices (openings).
- Brushing your teeth less than two hours prior to oral sex
- Brushing your teeth can cause tiny cuts in your mouth.
- Oral secretions can transmit (HIV, Herpes, Syphilis, Hepatitis B, and Genital Warts).
- Sharing sheets, underwear, towels, and bathing suits
- This can lead to the transfer of Crabs, Scabies, Body Lice, and Trichomoniasis.
- Rubbing or massaging your partner's skin
- If the person has open sores or rashes and you touch them, you may catch Syphilis or Cancroids.

- Rubbing naked bodies together or dry humping with clothes off can lead to the transmission of skin related disease.
- Hand job or masturbation
- If you are touching your partner's penis or external female genitals and he or she is infected with Syphilis, Herpes, Hepatitis, Crabs, Scabies, Genital Warts or MRSA, you could become infected as well.
- Putting your finger in the vagina or rectum
- You could catch Chlamydia, Gonorrhea, Yeast Infection, Bacterial Vaginosis (BV), Scabies, or Crabs.
- Performing oral sex
- Generally oral sex is safe if there is no exchange of semen or pre-cum, blood, or vaginal secretions. If any of these fluids are present, you're at risk of every STD I mentioned under this category.

Moderate Risk:

- Vaginal or anal sex
- These two natural orifices can transmit any STD found around the opening, even with a condom.
- Putting one or more digits (fingers) in your partner's vagina or anus can open up microscopic sores, cuts, and lesions. This could expose you to STDs, HIV, Herpes, Hepatitis, Nongonococcal Specific Urethritis (NSU), Scabies, Crabs or Genital Warts.
- Sharing dildos or sex toys with the purpose of penetration can transfer infectious fluids.
- If the sex device comes in contact with fluids, secretions, sores, warts, bumps, or open wounds, you could catch numerous STDs, HIV, Hepatitis, Herpes, Scabies and or Crabs. Sharing means each partner is penetrating the other without disinfecting the device between uses.

High Risk:

- Oral sex or rimming (oral/anal sex)
- Contact to these areas with your mouth without a condom or dental dam can result in disease exposure. You could catch any STD's, skin infections, immune disorder diseases, Hepatitis (Liver Disease), and Parasites.
- Vaginal or anal intercourse
- Penetration with either of these two natural orifices without a condom or latex barrier can expose you to secretions that can transmit disease.
- Sharing needles
- All blood-borne diseases can be transmitted from a surgical needle if the presence of even a small amount of blood is left in the bevel of the needle or syringe.

This is how educational awareness begins. These categories and the behavior associated with each will help you in your decision-making process evaluating whether you should continue at the level of risk you are currently at; they may also persuade you to think twice before elevating your sexual behavior to the next level. Regardless of the sexual behavior you decide to engage in, talk it over with your partner. He or she may have a very different set of morals related to sexual activity.

There is a full gamut of personal and professional protective equipment that can be utilized by anyone. All items are readily available, reasonably priced, and easy to use. Everything from protective hand gloves to condoms and everything in between have been demonstrated to decrease any chance or opportunity to come in contact with bodily fluids that can harm you.

Regardless of the behavior or type of exposure you are having with any individual, you have to make a responsible decision for yourself.

Do you need to protect yourself, or should you gamble on your own impulse? The choice is yours.

Occupational risks are slightly different and harder to control. Protection requires constant awareness of your work surroundings, understanding the professional tasks that pose a risk, and identifying through the educational and training process the steps you can take to protect yourself from those risks.

If you work in a profession where the job task you are trained to perform as a normal routine has the potential of exposure to bodily fluids or secretions, the Occupational Health and Safety Administration (Federal and State OSHA) requires your employer to have in place a written occupational exposure control plan. The plan must include the type of tasks that could lead to exposure, steps the employee can take to modify that behavior to avoid contact to potentially infectious agents, pre- and post-exposure decontamination procedures, reporting and documentation forms, and steps you can take to be tested and treated if necessary. Lastly, the exposure control plan will include a list of the personal protective equipment you should use to eliminate contact of someone else's body fluids to your skin or natural openings.

Although your employer may have fulfilled his or her legal obligation to protect employees, it's imperative that you exercise universal precautions under any circumstances. Treat everyone and all bodily fluids as potentially infectious. The protective barriers that you should have access to include but are not limited to: eye protection, safety gloves, rescue breathing masks (CPR/FA), protective outerwear, respirators (if applicable), and disinfectants.

For the purpose of demonstration, we will start with eye protection. This often consists of safety goggles, which should always be clear not tinted, manufactured with brow and side guards that will prevent any sweat and another person's respiratory secretions (coughing or sneezing) from entering your eyes. Eye protection usually is one-size-fits-all and can be cleaned for reuse.

Hand gloves must also be provided to all employees at all times. The material that provides the greatest protection factor currently is nitrile, followed by 100 percent latex. Both materials have demonstrated a protection factor of 97.2 percent to 99.5 percent. This means that if you bought a box of one hundred pairs of gloves, maybe two or three pairs would not protect you from possible infection. Two factors considered in the failure rating are: 1) the misuse of the product, and 2) faulty manufacturing. All protective gloves should be available to you in different sizes (small, large, and extra large). This is to prevent the tearing of the material when putting them on, pressure points that make the material thinner, or being so large that they slip off when in use. All hand protection wear is for one use only and should be discarded appropriately. The only exception to this rule is Kevlar gloves, which are puncture and cut resistant. If cleaned and stored according to manufacturers' guidelines, they should last approximately twenty-five years.

What is startling to me every time I pick up a newspaper, read a magazine, or listen to headline news, is that the number of cases of infectious disease carriers and outbreaks continues to rise every day. Every time a new product comes on the market that has been designed and tested and is specific in use, there is always some type of controversy or conflict as to the effectiveness of the product. For instance, condoms, which come in many different styles and materials, have continued to be misused due to the lack of understanding of the application process and how it protects you.

For years, lambskin condoms were the condom of choice; they were considered at that time to be the safest and most effective to prevent pregnancy and the transmission of disease. Long-term research has now indicated that, at best, lambskin condoms have only a 60 percent protection factor. Compare that to modern-day latex condoms, which have been proven to have a success rate and protection factor of between 97.2 percent and 99.5 percent. If you do the math, this would indicate that by using latex products, you have a greater than 30 percent chance of protecting yourself from pregnancy or being infected with a potentially life-threatening disease. Could there be products on the markets that are safer than the traditional latex condom? Currently, Japanese scientists are working with a material that is 55 percent thinner than current condoms and increase the sensitivity, protection from pregnancy and disease.

Understand there are no 100-percent guarantees with any products. Many times we actually make the conscientious decision to buy protective barriers and then either misuse them or don't use them at all when needed. An example of this is when you are under the influence of drugs or alcohol, both of which impair your decision-making process. Other factors that prevent you from applying the condom you took the time to buy may be the pressures of not knowing how to use it correctly, or because of the heat of the moment, both of you overlook the possible risk you are taking choosing passion over prevention of pregnancy or disease.

The size of the condom you choose and how you use it will determine the level of safety you have provided yourself and your partner. Like other parts of our body, the genitalia grow to different sizes. There is no such thing as a one-size-fits-all condom. Obviously, condoms are manufactured and sold in different sizes. Manufacturers of these prophylactic barriers realized that even with the increase in sales, there still was a concern that due to the lack of education, these barriers were being misused because of labeling flaws and the introduction of flavors and ribbed and texture options.

The greatest concern regarding the misuse of condoms is that a man will, due to his own ego, try to accommodate himself using a prophylaxis that is too large. The possibility of it slipping off, with semen and sperm dripping down the collar of the condom, will obviously increase the chances of his partner being impregnated or infected. Having recognized this, the manufacturing companies no longer label condoms as small, medium, large, or extra large. The industry joke is, "What man in his right mind would go into a local pharmacy and ask for a box of small condoms with ten women standing behind him in line?" *None*, obviously! Manufacturers of condoms now label them differently, such as magnum, super magnum, or my favorite, "not in my lifetime magnum."

In 1992, manufacturers in the US and Europe with the approval from the FDA and European Medicine Agency (EMA), marketed the first female condom. It is known, of course, that there are many women who prefer not to use male condoms because of the loss of sensitivity and the issue of spontaneity during the sexual act itself. The female condom provides a new direction in self-protection. The female condom, if you are not aware, is a thin sheath or pouch worn by the woman during intercourse. It completely lines the vagina and uterus and helps to protect from pregnancy and STDs. There are two types of female condoms available; one termed the FC and the other the FC2, female and male condom. The FC female condom has been available in Europe since its inception in 1992. This product was tested and approved by the US Food and Drug Administration that same year. It took forty to sixty million dollars in research to determine the level of safety required by the FDA to protect the user from infectious disease or pregnancy. Now, I don't know about you, but I didn't realize there was a difference between European women and American women as it relates to their anatomy. So why did it take millions of dollars in research to come to the same conclusion?

This product comes in limited quantities unfortunately throughout the world. The price of this product is expensive, which can be a deterrent. Here in the United States, the brand names go unrecognized and are not advertised. In other countries, you would discover names like

Reality, Femdom, Domonique, Femy, My Femy, Protective, and Care. The largest manufacturer of these products is Avert.

One downside to the female condoms is it's only six and a half inches in length. This may not fully protect a woman who has an enlarged uterus or vaginal opening. Other disadvantages are that the outer ring is visible outside the vagina, which makes some women self-conscious in front of their partners. The condom itself makes a crackling and popping noise during intercourse. Experts advise the user to apply more lubrication to lessen the noise. The female condom has a higher failure rate than non-barrier methods, such as oral contraceptive pills. The birth control pill, in return, however, won't prevent STDs. The female condom is somewhat cumbersome to insert and is for one use. The average price prevents teens from purchasing them because of the expense.

The advantages of using the female condom are many, however. When a man penetrates the vaginal opening of the woman, the condom naturally unravels to accommodate the male penis. A situation that often occurs before or during sex is that the male decides in the heat of the moment that he doesn't want to interrupt the passion and take the time to put a condom on. So the female has the option to use the female condom, especially if she isn't using any other form of protection. The polyurethane is less likely to cause an allergic reaction than a male latex condom. The female condom is sold over the counter without a prescription, unlike a diaphragm; and it does not need to be fitted by a medical provider (one size truly does fit all in this case), another advantage over the male condom.

The female condom will protect the user from sexually transmitted infections (STI) and sexually transmitted diseases (STD), if it is used correctly. The difference between an STI and a STD is that the latter develops into a systemic condition verses just a symptom. These female condoms also can cover the vulva for added protection. The outer ring can stimulate the clitoris during intercourse, and allows for tongue insertion and fingering of the vagina or anus. Just one piece of advice: if using the female condom for anal penetration, remove the inner ring before insertion. Lastly, the female condom can be inserted up to eight hours prior to sex, so it doesn't interfere with the moment. You can go on a number of websites to educate yourself in the use of these condoms. On a positive note, unlike the male condom, female condoms have much longer shelf life expectancy, up to three years versus a one-year maximum for the male condom. They also have very few storage requirements and may be used with numerous types of lubricants. The question that has been asked many times is, "What if you have sensitivity or an allergic reaction to latex materials like male condoms?" Good news, the female condom is manufactured using nitrol, which is what most hand gloves are made of today. On a final note, the female condom has been demonstrated to have a 1 percent failure rate, according to all manufacturers on these products.

The World Health Organization's primary concern is that in poverty-stricken areas of the world, the expense of these condoms causes nearly 30 percent of all individuals who purchase and use these condoms to simply wash them out in a household sink for reuse. Multiple use of the same condom could result in a faulty, non-protective product, which when not cleaned properly may still harbor microorganisms and pathogens that carry disease. The recommendation is that it be used only once, which was issued by the manufacturer's specifications along with the findings of the FDA approval committee. Scientific proof has shown that certain diseases can exist in these barriers for not just hours but even days. Remember, protective barriers are one of three layers of defense against disease. Your skin is the first and your second being your own immune system. If either is disrupted or comes in contact with a potentially infected bodily fluid, disease transmission may occur. This information, hopefully, will give you the awareness of how to protect yourself against disease and unwanted pregnancy.

Unfortunately, the use of condoms has now decreased because of the complacency and naivety in this 21ˢᵗ Century era of teenagers. In fact, promiscuous behavior has increased significantly over the past few years globally. These statistics are alarming and at the same time not heavily documented or reported by the media. An example: The microorganisms Chlamydia, Gonorrhea, Syphilis, Herpes and Vaginosis accounted for 1.5 million infections just in America according to the CDC 2008 statistic reports. Many of these cases go undiagnosed or unreported. Then we can add to that HIV/AIDS and HPV, which is of particular concern to the scientific community. These statistics combined, currently make up 3.2 million cases in North America.

African men and woman carry the biggest burden in the world today. Some villages have reported a 100 percent infected rate to HIV which would indicate that every boy, girl, husband and wife, grandmother and grandfather, and every baby being born today in that village is a carrier of HIV. According to the World Health Organization surveillance report 2009 and SOS Foundation account have conclusively determined there is an epidemic of AIDS that impact every country, city and village in Africa with an estimated total of 22.5 million carriers. A portion of Africa called the Sub-Saharan African region has an estimated 40 percent of the work aged population has contracted HIV, with younger and more successful workers most likely infected as well. In addition to these risk groups, when you add females, pregnant lactating mothers and infants being born with HIV, means there are areas where virtually everyone has contracted HIV/AIDS.

The worst effected countries are Swaziland, Botswana, Zimbabwe and Lesotho. In countries like these, they have no young adults left uninfected. The CDC and the World Health Organization didn't expect that type of devastating statistic for another ten to twenty years.

Reducing the preventable and persistent toll of STDs and other diseases will require expanding access to, not just protective barriers, but also prevention and treatment coupled with screening services for everyone.

What is interesting is that humans collectively have the desire, the need, and the willingness to feel intimate and loved and to be sexually active. So, at some point in our lifetime, we are going to experience some type of social interaction, intimate contact, or indiscreet relations with another person that could place you at risk. Abstinence is the only way to prevention.

Condoms, whether for men or women, can only live up to the standards of protection the manufacturers strive for if their customers are using them correctly and in combination with other forms of protection, such as dental dams, finger cots, and plastic wrap. Just in case you're not familiar with these terms or devices, I will define each, the purpose for using it, the protection factor, and steps to use it safely and effectively.

Dental dams are a byproduct of the homosexual community. This prophylactic barrier was manufactured decades ago for the dental industry. Its original design was to protect the patient from any flying debris from the mouth while extracting teeth, root canals, crowns, and bridgework, or simply when drilling into a tooth to remove a cavity. It is made of 100 percent latex, comes in different sizes, is applied by the dental assistant or doctor over the patient's entire mouth, and is secured to the tooth to be worked on by a clamp. The advantage to both the patient and dentist is that no exchange of body fluid or secretions as well as tooth particles can occur if applied correctly.

You're probably asking yourself what this has to do with sex in the gay community. Back in the mid to late 1980s, I was conducting a training seminar in Los Angeles, California. During my class, I was approached by an individual who mentioned he was partnered with the Gay and Lesbian Community Outreach Program in Garden Grove, a city just south of LA. He said that even though my seminar was informative, the information followed the same mainstream educational process that government agencies alerting the public of emerging health risks wanted all educators to follow. At this time, the immediate crisis was from a mysterious disease that was causing tremendous illness and death to young gay men. Later this disease was formally identified as HTLV3 or, as its known today, HIV.

He invited me to be his guest at one of his seminars and critique his approach to the information they were presenting to gays and lesbians. I was thinking, *how different could this possibly be?* We already know that no disease discriminates based on sexual origin or any other physical parameters. But I went with an open mind.

After the usual introduction to different types of sexual behavior and the health risks that could follow, he began a section on personal protective barriers. To my surprise, I learned something new. The homosexual community had become very creative in ways they could continue on with a "normal sexual relationship" and at the same time protect themselves from the novel virus HIV. So they introduced and experimented with a device called a dental dam, and damn if he wasn't right. The dental dam is made of the same protective material used in condoms, which is 100 percent latex. This medical material can be purchased at most medical and dental supply stores, and you don't have to be a doctor or dentist to purchase it.

The manufacturers caught word of this extracurricular use of the dams and got creative themselves. The dams are now made in different widths and lengths, colors and flavors. Have you ever put a latex glove in your mouth? It wasn't too pleasant, I'm sure. Some individuals have allergies to latex material, so the dams are also made from nitrol. This reduces the chances for any sensitive reaction to the skin.

The technique for applying the dental dam can be a bit awkward and time-consuming, just like a condom.

To avoid any contact to the genitals and body fluids from your partner, place the dam on the genitals to be stimulated and then place your mouth and tongue over the dam and apply force for stimulation. These devices can be bought for hands-free use. Just place the material between two specially designed head straps and tighten. Now your hands are free to excite other parts of your partner's body at the same time. After use, discard the dental dam, as you would a condom. Remember, it's for one use only.

Another device being used for the purpose of protection is finger cots. The sexual activity is digital sex (fingering). Finger cots are used frequently by OB/GYN doctors as well as dentists. They prevent the necessity of using an entire prophylactic barrier. The finger cot covers just the first or second knuckle of the finger. When you are performing sexual penetration using just your fingers, consider using the finger cot. The protection factor is the same as condoms and dental dams. They are manufactured using latex or nitrol, which provide a 99.2 percent to 99.7 percent protection from disease present in all bodily fluids, including blood. Tattoo artists also use finger cots for protection and greater hand control of the ink injector and for dexterity.

One more technique that is considered by many as a protective barrier against STDs and is widely used as birth control is vaginal douching. If this procedure is your go-to technique for either of these reasons, you seriously need to read on. According to CDC, NIH, WHO, and dozens if not hundreds of other researchers and manufactures of douching products indicate these could make your situation worse. If you remember back in the early 1980s (a lot of reminiscing in this book), there was a television commercial that featured a daughter asking her mom, "Do you ever get that not-so-fresh smell?" The advertisement was for a brand of douche, a feminine hygiene product for women to use to clean their vagina. According to the website, www.womenshealth.gov, it is now estimated that 20 to 40 percent of American women 15 to 44 years old douche regularly. They use a douche to clean the vagina, rinse away blood after monthly periods, get rid of odor, avoid sexually transmitted infections (STIs) and/or prevent pregnancy.

Yet health experts say douching isn't effective for all of these purposes. They actually warn the consumer that it could increase the risk of infections, pregnancy complications, and other health problems. Overall, the risks of douching far outweigh the benefits. Douching has been found to disrupt the normal balance of bacteria in the vagina (called vaginal flora). These changes of the concentration of good bacteria will allow the growth of bad bacterium to develop in the vaginal cavity that may cause infection. Studies have shown that women who stop douching are less prone to bacterial vaginosis (BV). A woman having BV increases her risk of a possible pre-term labor and endometriosis. According to the women health website mentioned above, state those women who douche have a greater than 75 percent chance for Pelvic Inflammatory Disease (PID). This can lead to other complications, such as cervical cancer or ectopic pregnancy, when the embryo implants itself outside the uterus, fallopian tubes, and ovaries.

The American College of Obstetricians and Gynecologists (ACOG), report that woman of all ages should avoid douching. The complications don't justify the simple purpose to eliminate an odor that is normal. Strong odors, however, may be a result of a major infection, which you should take care of immediately with a visit to your OB/GYN. As an alternative, just wash the area with warm water and soap. The acidity of the vagina will naturally control bacteria.

Always weigh the pros and cons before submitting to any medical or hygienic procedure, and be very observant of the techniques and protection your doctor is using on you.

I recently went through surgery myself and was extremely cautious of the sterile procedures the nurses, doctors, and surgeons were implementing prior to the procedure. That is until the morphine and anesthesia kicked in, and then I was at their mercy. The medical staff attends hours of training to prepare them for aseptic techniques and procedures. Yet we continue to see an increase in the number of cases of disease (especially skin infections like MRSA) at these facilities, which should be sterile and immune to these illness-causing invaders.

The problem is obvious. Without the presence of human beings, they could achieve their goals. The patients coming in off the street cross-contaminate every surface they touch. We must rely on the technology and safe practices our medical care personnel have been taught, instructing them how to use personal protective equipment (PPE) when having contact with their patients.

Keep in mind that you can utilize any one of the protective barriers we've been reviewing in this chapter, but you still may be at risk of disease, especially airborne illnesses, just by breathing. The environment is your greatest risk at this point. So unless you're in a sterile (not just clean) environment, you're never fully immune to disease.

In review, we have discovered many different techniques and protective barriers you should always use during sexual relations. I know that at times this impacts the spontaneity of the moment, the application may be awkward at first (everyone gets better with practice), and the costs may seem unaffordable, especially if you're extremely active sexually. But how do you put a dollar amount on your health, safety, and life? Don't put yourself and others at risk of disease. These diseases are always present and constantly changing so they can crash your party.

CHAPTER 7
IS OUR GOVERNMENT KEEPING US SICK? SCREENING AND TESTING

When comparing this chapter to those in the rest of this book, we have to bring into question the motives of the Centers for Disease Control and Prevention, National Association of Infectious Diseases, Food and Drug Administration, World Health Organization, and many other public health and safety agencies. Are these agencies truly fulfilling their legal and moral obligations to protect the citizens of the United States and human beings worldwide? Voluntary and mandatory testing haven't changed much since the discovery of new diseases that have decimated whole societies and created fear, discontent, and the feeling of hopelessness for millions of people around the globe. Is it unfair to ask the scientists and health officials who discover these new or ongoing potentially life-threatening conditions to properly inform citizens in those areas directly impacted by the outbreaks and allow access to medical screening, testing, and the appropriate treatment to impact the health consequences they are suffering from? Most of the regions are experiencing plagues, epidemics, mini pandemics, famine, and sanitary conditions that are more degrading than the living conditions in our city zoos.

The World Health Organization (WHO) is not there to help with humanitarian needs these regions rightly deserve. It is also my opinion that the FDA and WHO are not fulfilling their obligations to supply towns, villages, and cities the medicines that are necessary to treat their conditions and prolong life. Screening and testing is not afforded to them, so many people already infected as carriers but not showing signs or symptoms of the disease are passing it on to other family members and anyone they have intimate contact with, not realizing it. As I mentioned earlier in the book, there are villages in Africa that have 100 percent infection rates. That means every person living in that village is infected with, in this case, HIV/AIDS.

This can be avoided with aggressive action from the agencies I listed above. However, these agencies plead poverty and state they don't have the manpower, money, or medical supplies necessary to eradicate these health problems being reported for years. What could we expect from these health officials if such problems were to occur here in the United States? History has already demonstrated that natural or man-made pandemics are possible anytime anywhere.

We must take matters in our own hands. Stop waiting for those health alerts before you finally take action. Be proactive with your life and health. Preventive medicine is one of the most important elements in breaking the chain of disease.

People approach me all the time about alternative testing for these diseases. There are other tests that can be done using other bodily fluids and secretions other then blood. We can test your urine, saliva, breast milk, vaginal secretions and even spinal fluid. These tests are only conducted in medical offices.

Whether you get tested or not, you have other options to help prevent infection or treat conditions related to infections and disease. The two practices are called Naturopathic and Alternative Medicine. These unorthodox means to prevent and/or treat disease processes have been around since the early 1900's. The two have nearly the same philosophy and beliefs in the success each system has achieved and evidence based results. They have demonstrated with many patients that vitalism, which relies on vital energy or a force that guides your entire being (both mental and physical) to achieve relief with pain, boost immune response and extend good health. The most efficient and safest way to increase immunity to disease is to eliminate everything that suppresses or weakens your body's defense sytem.

I occasionally infuse into my speaking seminars jokes or light hearted candor with different topics. In the case of strengthening your immune system, I casually mention that you can accomplish this simply by avoiding that morning coffee and add an orange to your diet. It also has been proven that caffeine has a negative effect on your immune system and the fruit that contain vitamin C and other vitamins will increase antibody production.

Here are a few examples of alternative approaches to better health:

1. Acupuncture
2. Chiropractic
3. Herbalism
4. Homeopathy
5. Energy Therapy
6. Manipulative Therapy
7. Meditation

Both Naturopathic (holistic) and Alternative Medicine (vitalism) try to find the least invasive procedures for symptom improvement and resolution, which is the entire premise of this book. By educating you and creating awareness of the risk factors that can lead to disease transmission in combination with providing you the tools and resources to protect yourself from exposure, I've accomplished the same thing. No drugs needed!! What was once considered taboo practices, are now growing collaborative efforts between naturopaths and medical doctors. There goal is to evaluate the safety and efficiency of Naturopathic and Alternative Medicine in prevention and management of a broad rang of ailments.Medical committees are also trying to decide whether accessibility of naturopathic services will enhance patient's health in a cost effective way. I am still a believer that the mind is stronger than our physical being. That follows the old passage "mind over matter".

When it comes to cost effectiveness, you can't argue that main stream medicine which includes but not limited to : surgery, physical therapy, pain relief practices, drugs, testing and follow-up care, far exceeds the costs of Naturopathic or Alternative Medicine practices.

 Through the education and awareness process in this book, we have learned to identify health risks that have occurred in our past, as well as those that impact our present and may evolve in our future. We have identified environments that harbor disease-causing microbes, behavior that can lead to direct and indirect contact with these organisms, the avenues by which they can enter your body and make you a new host for that particular disease, and finally, once such an organism is in your system, the illnesses and complications that can cause death.

When we concluded Chapter 3 with the final link in the chain of transmission, I left you wondering, if you were involved in a situation where all four links in the chain of transmission were present at the time of exposure and the microorganism somehow gained access to your bloodstream, would you know this had just happened to you? If I remember correctly, I joked that you might wake up the next morning with a burden of weight to one side of your body, as if this microscopic organism contained that much mass, or that you might suddenly feel a sharp pain, let's say, in one of your arms or legs.

Well, it doesn't work that way. There are only two indicators that you are a carrier of any disease, and they are:

1. You begin to show signs and symptoms of an illness.
2. You get tested, and your results indicate the presence of a disease in your system. The reason why I did not say you tested positive or negative is because the results could be a false positive or false negative. I will explain below how this happens.

The reason for continual testing is to identify possible carriers of disease to prevent further spreading of their infections to others. Most people, however, choose not to get tested because they are afraid the results may return positive. The psychological effect that comes with bad news is obvious. Questions you may begin to ask yourself include: Do I share this information with my family or closest friends? Are they going to judge me for being infected? It reminds me of the scarlet letter pinned on the chest of carriers with scarlet fever (the big S). They had to wear it anytime they were in public, with the victim usually scorned to the point of suicide. I don't recall in this society the scarlet letter H (HIV) being worn by anyone—or STD, HPV, TB, or MRSA monikers. Your test results are always kept confidential and are only reported to the health department by age, sex, gender, and county or state for statistical reasons. Don't hesitate to get tested for any disease you are suspicious of or that you think you were possibly exposed to.

Since I worked for many years in the medical field dealing with patient care, usually in extreme acute care scenarios, I always have taken the responsible road to test twice a year for many of the diseases mentioned earlier. The sooner I know my true status, the better. If it happens to come back positive, I can immediately begin the steps I need to take to fight the disease, stay healthier longer, and not put anyone else at risk. I can also sleep better at night knowing I'm negative. You should consider this same approach. No one is going to come banging on your door to get you tested.

Situations that may require you to submit to disease screening or testing are as follows:

1. Anyone accused of physical assault or rape.
2. Intake process for high-risk offenders for the purpose of incarceration.
3. Donated blood is always screened for certain diseases.
4. You are required to submit to testing in order to receive a life insurance policy.
5. Unique occupations, such as tattoo artist, pornography actor, phlebotomist (if you have experienced a needle stick).
6. A court order signed by a judge ordering testing.

In to many situations, a person who may be concerned about their disease status and should have themselves tested for sexual acquired infections, hesitate or refuse to test for a few reasons. First, this individual may be afraid of receiving a positive test result, which will confirm their status as a carrier. These results could impact that person both emotionally and physically. Seeing and hearing the results (if positive) immediately consumes your brain with thoughts of doom and gloom. The consequences are unknown at first and depending on which disease(s) you are now a host of, will change your life forever.

Second, it is apparent that even time cannot shake the stereotypic opinion of the uneducated public about diseases such as HIV/AIDS. Since the very first case reported back in the late 1970's, this disease is still considered primarily a homosexual disease. The fact is HIV infection among homosexuals has leveled off and in a few subcategories actually has declined. Other risk groups that are on the rise are the heterosexual community and IV drug users.

The injustice that occurs when you don't get screened or tested, delays treatment that could slow down the disease process that could extend you life, but also may be the catalyst for you to spread the disease to other partners in the future without realizing it. If you don't know you're infected, how could anyone else. The most recent surveys conducted by many reputable reporting agencies indicated that nearly 30 percent of newly tested participants whose blood test came back positive for the HIV antibodies, could not determine how they got the disease. They also could not identify the behavior (contact) that led to the transmission or identify which person gave them the virus.

After nearly three decades of its presence here in North America, we are no closer to finding a cure or vaccine for HIV. In fact, the virus is changing, adapting faster and more effectively inside the human host than anticipated. For those reasons, the scientific community is actually going backwards in HIV research.

So, do yourself and others a great service and get tested.

If you're concerned that your privacy will not be protected from information that could be shared with other parties, you have a valid reason to think that way. However, the privacy laws have changed to protect those individuals that chose to be screened and tested.

In the worst case scenario, you go to your private doctor and he/she suggest that you get tested for an STD. Your name is then kept confidential and you're assigned a case number. The only down side is that your test results will be placed in your medical records. Although that information is confidential, there are some situations that will allow other parties to legally gain access to your test results.

For instance, you are applying for a life insurance policy for an exceptionally high value, your insurer can ask for any and all test results as it relates to STD's including Hepatitis and HIV. If you have yet to be tested, they may require you to submit to testing before they would issue a policy. Secondly, if you have been accused of committing a sexual crime, the Judge in charge of your case could order a bench warrant to confirm your disease status. If you still refuse at that point, the court could hold you in contempt.

To avoid all the confusion, misconceptions and fears with testing, the Food and Drug Administration (FDA) has given approval to a handful of companies that have developed home testing kits which will allow you to test yourself in the privacy of your own home.

The U.S. Center for Disease Control Hotline has all the information you would need to pursue home testing. The hotline is open 24 hours a day, 7 days a week at 1-800-CDC-INFO. Your other option is to visit the websites; I have listed below that provide the FDA approved home testing kits.

1. www.thebody.com: They provide anonymous testing to determine your level of risk to HIV.
2. www.homehealthtesting.com: This Company has developed and sells Express HIV-1 tests which are 99 percent accurate. They take privacy issues very seriously, so they mail the home testing kit to the address of your choice in a plain paper box with a return address of MLSC, Inc. there parent company. You register to receive your results using a unique code number.
3. www.stdalert.com: STD Alert has received FDA approval with ten of its home testing products. These would include, Chlamydia, Gonorrhea, Herpes I, Herpes II, HIV I & HIV II, Hepatitis A, B, C and Syphilis. The company also has DNA testing for HIV, not just the Elisa/Western Blot test that identifies the antibodies developed by your immune response to the virus that now exists in your blood stream.

When you experience a situation that makes you concerned about your own status, meaning you came in contact with someone else's bodily fluids or secretions, you need to get tested to determine if you were infected as a direct result of that situation.

Let's say you went out last night with your friends to a social gathering in which drugs and alcohol was involved. The liquid courage kicked in, and you started having a conversation with someone you had never met before. Before you realized it, he or she was inviting you back to his or her place for a nightcap. Soon the conversation got more intimate, and before you realized it, you ended up having sex with this person without proper protection.

So, you woke up the next morning and proceeded home to shower. As you begin to review what happened that night, you start feeling a bit concerned that something could have happened during your physical time together. You don't feel sick, and there are no signs that you caught an infection. You're concerned enough, however, that you decide to call your doctor and set up an appointment to come in for an evaluation and possible testing to be safe.

Remember that all disease has an incubation or window period where there won't be enough bacterial or viral loading to be detectable and your immune system hasn't created the antibodies to fight against the disease. So your first test will most likely come back negative. You would then have to follow up in the next month or two and submit to a confirmatory test. This will prove the first test to be a false negative if the current results come back positive. If the results are still negative, you have a 98 percent chance that the two negative tests are true negative.

Let's say the disease you were most concerned about was HIV and that was the test you submitted to. The name of this test is HIV ELISA/Western Blot. It consists of a simple blood test and takes about seven to ten days to get the results. No preparation, such as fasting or drinking any strange medical liquid, is necessary. After the test is conducted, if the results come back positive, a western blot test is always given. A positive Western Blot confirms an HIV infection. If the Western Blot is negative, it means the HIV ELISA test was false positive. The western blot test can also be unclear, in which case more testing will be necessary.

When the scientific community tries to determine the average incubation or "window" period for all disease that can be identified through testing, we first must determine the approximate time period in which you were involved in a behavior that reasonably could have led to the transmission. That's why it is so important for you not to wait to get tested; we don't want you exposed in another way to the disease we are testing for, which gives us a better chance of identifying the person who was a carrier of the same disease and what the exact contact was that allowed for the transfer of the disease from his or her system to yours.

If you test negative to the antibodies, we will have you retest in three months, six months, nine months, and twelve months and then twice a year after the original test date. Tests will be required at this rate until your results convert to serum positive. For HIV, the average incubation currently is six months to two years. This incubation period occurs with 96 percent of all cases. If you notice, there still is 4 percent missing. Studies indicate that 1 percent of all cases will test positive within three months after exposure, with the last 3 percent testing positive for the antibodies as long as ten years after infection.

Another test often asked for is Hepatitis A, B, and C. This test is similar to the HIV test; it consists of a blood sample. All of these tests are referred to as baseline results. That way when you follow up with a confirmatory test, the medical doctor has something to compare it to. Surveillance of your blood counts can also indicate other infections you didn't test for initially. The incubation periods for Hepatitis disease range from two to eighteen months, 99 percent of the time. Approximately 1 percent of individuals tested may take as long as two years or more to convert positive.

Tuberculosis (TB) fortunately can be detected much more quickly. The test universally used for TB detection is called the Purified Protein Derivative (PPD) skin test. This test is also referred to as the Mantoux tuberculin sensitivity test. This is just one of two major skin tests that replaced the multi-puncture test called the Tine test. A dose of five Tuberculin units (0.1mL) is injected intradermal (between the layers of the skin), forming a small bubble under the skin that dissipates quickly. The patient will be asked to return for a skin reaction reading forty-eight to seventy-two hours later. A person who has been exposed to the bacteria is expected to mount an immune response at the injection site containing bacterial proteins. The injection is given on the forearm. If a positive reaction occurs, the skin will be raised and hardened. The medical practitioner will measure the reactive area in millimeters.

Once you test positive, your PPD results will always test positive. This simply indicates that you were at some point in your life exposed to active TB disease. There is no need to worry at this point because as long as you're not sick or symptomatic, you're non-infectious to others. The disease can lie dormant in your body for months, years, and even decades without causing an illness. The bacteria, however, may become active just because of subtle changes in your health or diet, drastic weight changes, or other diseases that compromise your immune system, such as HIV, Diabetes, and Cancers. Medical treatments like chemotherapy, radiation, and dialysis also may activate TB disease.

After testing with the conventional skin tests, if the medical officer in charge of your case is still suspicious of your true status, you can also be tested for the bacterium using throat cultures, tissue biopsies, and chest X-rays. These tests can also be used as confirmatory tests for the PPD skin results. Tuberculosis is a respiratory disease that can only be spread from one host to another when it is active and present in your airway passages or lungs. Just coughing, laughing, or sneezing will allow the bacterium to become airborne by piggybacking on your respiratory molecules. Then the people that are in close proximity to you simply inhale those infected particles into their lungs. Infections that are caused by airborne pathogens are far more difficult to trace the source host than diseases that are transmitted by means of intimate contact or body fluids and secretions.

Sexually Transmitted Diseases (STDs), Sexually Transmitted Infections (STI), and Venereal Diseases (VD) can be transmitted numerous ways, including indirect contact. There is a wide range of sexually transmitted disease tests that can be conducted for you, but first you must inform your health-care provider of any sexual activity you have engaged in with your partner(s) to give a better understanding of which disease(s) you might have caught because of those actions. The world of STDs is comprised of many different forms of pathogens. They could be Bacteria, Fungi, Viral, Parasites, or Protozoal in nature. If the disease is bacterial, this may include Chancroid, Chlamydia, Gonorrhea, and Syphilis. Fungal infections would include Candidiasis (yeast infection). Viral infections include Hepatitis A, B, C, D, and E, Herpes Simplex and Human Papillomavirus are both viruses as well. Protozoal Infections are typically Trichomoniasis (vaginalis).

The testing for these different categories of STDs can be as simple as a urine or blood test or can involve fecal cultures or swabbing of the throat, penis, or vaginal area, especially if there are open sores, pus pockets, or discharge from those areas. All of these diseases have incubation periods and may go undetected for weeks or months without the carrier realizing he or she is infected, thereby possibly passing it on to future sexual partners. Just another reminder to always wear protection before sexual activity begins. One of my favorite sayings is, "Well, they look healthy." Looks, as we have found out, can be misleading.

Remember that repetitive engagement can double or triple your chances of being infected. This should send up a warning signal to get an initial screening and test for the diseases listed even if you're not currently ill. Preventive medicine helps you with early detection and prevents future behavior from spreading the infection to other partners. For better clarification Wikipedia has produced a chart which lists the odds of transmission per unprotected sexual act with an infected person. It indicates the sex acts, known risk and possible or unknown risks at:

(http://en.wikipedia.org/wiki/Sexually_transmitted_disease).

Let's put aside personal testing for a moment. Recently, California State Corrections Department and other state have been ordered by the Federal Government to enact an early release program for low-level prisoners back to the county jails. This has triggered and early release of jail inmates which is due to lean fiscal times. California, Colorado, Illinois, Kentucky, Michigan, Oregon and Wisconsin are among the states that have recently accelerated prisoner releases or are considering doing so according to the website www.newjerseynewsroom.com. and many other states are facing. The nation's budget crisis and Federal and State correctional system decline in funding have made it necessary. These actions will be in effect by 2012. One of the programs that had the greatest impact on releasing prisoners early was the cost of medical services provided to the inmates.

If you take into account the lack of testing while incarcerated and the fact that prisoners are not required to submitting to testing before their release back to the streets, you have the potential for a health catastrophe that could end up in your backyard. The Bureau of Justice Statistic Report by the U.S. Department of Justice, Office of Justice

Programs determined how many inmates at the State and Federal level were infected with Hepatitis A, B and C. If an inmate refused to have his or her blood drawn, the head of the state's correctional system got a judge to approve an injunction and blanket order for all inmates to submit to testing under the search warrant clause. In other words, they were approaching this disease as if it were a weapon. After the results were calculated, the study indicated that six in ten prisoners were infected with hepatitis. Once the prisoners have been released to the streets, independent states don't have the resources available to monitor their health, which could put the general public at risk.

It is estimated that the percentage of inmates infected could be as high as 82 percent because of the high-risk behavior they participate in while in prison, such as unprotected sex, tattoos, and physical altercations. These fights can lead to other inmates' exposure to blood and contribute to the high rates of infection. Poor hygienic practices with prisoners and facilities that are routinely cross-contaminated also result in an increase of disease carriers. This is the person who could end up being your daughter's next prom date, or the person who assaults you or invades your home.

When the issue of donated blood was addressed by the public and watchdog groups, the question of adequate testing is often the center point in the reports. Blood banks have a legal responsibility to screen donors prior to receiving their blood. That way we immediately eliminate them from the pool of donors potentially infected blood or plasma. The screening process begins with asking the right questions and identifying if the donor is telling the truth about his or her medical history.

In September 2006, the Food and Drug Administration fined the most reputable blood bank in the world, the American Red Cross (ARC), for $4.2 million for its failure to meet established blood-safety laws. ARC was fined mainly because it did not comply with an amended 2003 consent decree that called for significant financial penalties when the American Red Cross neglected to implement provisions designed to ensure the safety of the nation's blood supply. The FDA findings clearly indicated that ARC failed to ask appropriate donor screening questions and failed to follow manufacturers' testing protocols. The results of this could have led to serious health consequences. Since the entry of the 2003 consent decree and prior to this action, ARC had received seven letters and been assessed a total of $5.7 million in penalties.

In 1995, the president of the American Red Cross was participating in a television interview and was asked numerous questions on the subject of safety with the current blood supply. To make a long interview short, let me just comment on her response when she was asked, "Of all of the blood donated, screened, tested, and prepared for the purpose of infusing, how many samples still somehow make it through the entire process still infected with the virus HIV?" Knowing that she could not say that the blood was 100 percent safe, the director stated to the viewing audience that for every 60,000 pints of blood that is donated, they estimate that at least one of those samples is infected with the HIV virus and the disease could be given to someone else through infusing or dialysis.

Now that doesn't appear too bad. The odds of me receiving that one infected sample are slim to none. That statistic would not prevent me from receiving donated blood, especially in a medical emergency that could save my life. But those numbers are also deceiving. The ARC has on hand at any given moment a national reserve of donated blood of around 230,000 pints. What the president of ARC didn't mention is that 230,000 pints is only a two-day supply. What that indicates to me is that every two days, an average of 3.8 people is infected with HIV directly from the blood supply system. That calculates to be 13.3 people a week, 53.2 people per month or 638.4 people annually. How safe does the donated blood sound to you now? Is it still worth the risk? The risk is only to the recipient of a blood transfusion, not the giver.

The whole blood can also be manufactured into other blood products, which could increase the number of recipients of potentially infected samples. The only way you can clearly state that the sample is disease free would be to conduct DNA/RNA testing that would identify the virus, unlike the ELISA and western blot tests, which only identify the antibodies that have been created by your immune system and are now in your bloodstream attacking the microbe. As a final note, don't be afraid to get tested. Remember, ignorance is not bliss, and what you don't know can harm you.

CHAPTER 8
TO VACCINATE OR NOT TO VACCINATE? (IT'S YOUR DECISION.)

The issue of vaccination is approaching controversial levels we haven't seen since the first vaccine was created back in 1952 by Dr. Jonas Salk. Ironically, back around the turn of the century, immunity was achieved only during the infancy state. Infants continued to carry the mother's immunity to certain diseases until around the age of three. Back then, babies were often bombarded with polio and Smallpox Viruses. These infants didn't catch the disease because the mothers had passed on to them antibodies through breast-feeding.

According to the World Health Organization, in the late 19 Century the first initial vaccine to fight against the polio virus did not provide long term immunity. In 1950 a number of control measures were implemented and smallpox was eradicated in many areas in Europe and North America. On May 8, 1980, the WHO announced the world was free of small pox and recommended that all countries cease vaccinations. From the time of its discovery to 1980 the virus had claimed of 500,000,000 lives worldwide

The Polio Virus Vaccine was developed through painstaking research over the first half of the century. This is a good example of why I decided not to pursue a career in laboratory research. I simply don't have the patience for it. With the help of the March of Dimes and President Roosevelt, Dr. Salk had the resources to begin his research and a career studying immunology. He began his research on the Polio Virus while attending the University of Pittsburgh in 1947. His first discovery was the ability to grow the virus in a cell culture. Then he had to find a way to make the virus less infectious. In 1952, Salk was the first to develop a successful vaccine mixture of the three types of virus. He developed a chemical called Formalin that inactivated the entire virus. In 1954, massive clinical trials were done in the United States and Canada with dramatic results. The vaccine has been highly effective, with a 70 to 90 percent protection rate. Polio was nearly eradicated from the face of the earth. There has not been a single case caused by the wild virus since 1979.

Here is a timeline of more recent vaccine dicoveries since the inception of the polio vaccine.

In August 1960, Albert Sabin's live Polio Vaccine was recommended by the US surgeon general to be licensed. By 1963, all three types of polio were combined into one vaccine.

In 1968, Maurice Hilleman discovered the first vaccine for the new influenza A virus, Type A2, the Hong Kong strain that was causing widespread illness in that city. On a side note, Merck, which we now know as Merck Sharp & Dohm, manufactured 9 million doses of the vaccine.

In 1969, the Rubella vaccine was licensed. The vaccine was Maurice Hilleman's second profound discovery. A devastating Rubella pandemic developed during 1962 to 1965 in the United States that caused birth defects and congenital rubella syndrome to approximately twenty thousand babies. Tens of thousands of mothers had miscarriages or elected to have abortions.

In 1971, there was a multitude of breakthrough vaccines. Approved were Measles, Mumps, and Rubella Vaccine and combined MMR, licensed by Merck Pharmaceutical.

In 1981, the FDA approved a sophisticated plasma-derived Hepatitis B Vaccine. In 1986, a new recombinant vaccine replaced the original one because of the improved success rate, reduced side effects, and increased protection factor.

These are just a few of the many vaccines discovered since the inception of genetic engineering. One would think given these amazing advancements with vaccines, inoculations, and immunizations that the populace would embrace and receive these firewalls that protect our bodies from devastating diseases.

Vaccines provide us with the same immunity from natural infections without the consequences of true infection. Vaccines can be made using three different strategies or techniques. The first is to weaken the virus by cleansing or removing parts of its genetic makeup. The second strategy is to inactivate the virus completely, by removing its RNA or DNA. The third is to use only one part of the virus, utilizing one viral protein. Bacterial Vaccines work a little bit differently. To create these vaccines, the following protocol must be met:

- Use the sugar that coats the bacterial surface.
- Inactivate the bacterial toxin, which is harmful.
- Purify the bacterial proteins.

The above description is as lay term as possible to avoid confusing anyone. The controversy related to vaccines is about the safety that's built into them. We all know that everything comes with some degree of risk. But do the benefits in this case simply outweigh the side effects?

For years, parents have acquired a false sense of security since the inception of vaccinations, inoculations, and immunizations. Prior to even entering preschool, our children are bombarded with shots designed to protect them from common childhood diseases. Our hope is that after receiving a particular vaccine, your immune system will be fooled into thinking that it's been invaded by a particular virus, thereby creating the antibodies needed to destroy it or hold it hostage to prevent an illness or disease process from developing.

Remember what I mentioned earlier in the book: I am not, I repeat, *not* trying to persuade you with your decision-making process. I am merely the messenger who has compiled information to argue both sides. The information I choose to write is based on years of collaborative research by experts in their respective professions. This information is also based on test studies on both humans and animals. Laboratory findings and statistical information also were considered and reviewed for clarity, content, and accuracy. This information is not based on anyone's theories or speculative thinking. It is not my goal to change what you believe, think, or perceive to be true or accurate, regardless of your thoughts; I am just stating the facts.

Now that I have that disclaimer out of the way, let's continue.

You're probably asking yourself: How do these vaccines and drugs get approved, and who are the governing bodies? It all starts and ends with the US Food and Drug Administration (FDA). As I move forward in this chapter, it's only fair to inform you of your rights as a citizen of the United States of America. In this country, unlike many others around the globe, we have certain rights to either accept or deny the injection of a vaccine into our bodies. So take a step back for a moment and look at vaccinations in their simplest form. There doesn't appear to be any reason you shouldn't receive this vial of genetic material that claims it will give you immunity against the disease it was designed for. But looking deeper into this primitive, and to some degree barbaric, way to protect people from the pathogens that surround us, maybe there are other alternatives that achieve the same level of success. Let's find out together.

In 1905, the US Supreme Court gave itself the legal authority to allow state governments to pass laws requiring citizens to accept certain vaccines. Today all fifty states have enacted vaccine laws that require proof of vaccination for children who will be attending day care, elementary school, junior and high school, or college. Some high school students, along with their college counterparts, have reached the legal adult age of eighteen. They now have the same rights as adults to make their own life decisions, right? Not so fast. You see, they also must obey the laws of the land even as adults. The only difference is, when you are a minor, the physician must get parental consent before starting any medical procedure. All states, for instance, allow for medical exemption to vaccination, and forty-eight states allow a religious exemption, with eighteen states that allow for personal, philosophical, or conscientious belief exemptions to vaccinations. Many of our states require that students attending school receive three dozen doses of vaccines to create immunity from childhood diseases. That sounds like overkill to me.

Many of the vaccines these patients are receiving may be unnecessary. Except for the very young or the elderly, the rest of us have already developed a natural immunity to certain diseases in society and don't need to be vaccinated. The way you find out is through a simple blood test called a titer test. This screening of your blood is designed to identify the antibodies that have been developed by your immune response to kill invading microbes in your system. Titer tests are used widely to determine if vaccines have worked in creating sufficient antibody levels in your system to protect you as well. Here are some basic principles that will help you make the proper decision to vaccinate or not.

When you exercise your right to voluntary vaccination for yourself or your child, the state law has built-in legal requirements for enforcing these programs. School and health officials can recognize your legal right to refuse a vaccination. They also have the legal authority to exercise their right (not yours) to enforce and approve exemption for vaccination based on religious beliefs. But most schools will refuse attendance of unvaccinated children during confirmed outbreaks of certain diseases for a defined period of time. Just remember, nobody has the moral authority to force you or your child to be injected with a vaccine without your informed consent, and you have the same right to exercise exemptions to vaccination.

The National Childhood Vaccine Injury Act of 1986 directed all doctors and other vaccine providers to give you and your child the risks and complications of the vaccines in written form before injection. Just remember that all vaccines come with a laundry list of possible side effects and complications that may occur in only a few recipients. You should never agree to a vaccination, drug, or other product that claims to protect you without getting all the details of the risks. It's like getting a second or third opinion from doctors before going through with a medical procedure, which injections are. There must be attached to every vial an insert describing every reported reaction and precautions. You can also request this information to be sent to you by the state health department, or go to www.NVIC. org or www.NVICadvocacy.org for information and copies of the information inserts.

During my research, I was outraged to learn of a side-door legislative issue that had been submitted to and reviewed by numerous federal agencies. They included but were not limited to the National Guard and other military branches, Homeland Security representatives, and the office of the president of the United States. Without the voice of the people, the Department of Homeland Security, under the Presidential Directive (HSPD 10), stipulates the right to enforce martial law on any person residing within the borders of the United States, forcing him or her to submit to any vaccinations approved by the Food and Drug Administration (FDA). This law was signed by

President George Bush February 11, 2004 to combat a developing or existing pandemic.

The directive clearly outlines the government's right to enforce the law at its discretion to force all people to receive the injections. If you refuse to take the vaccine, state health personnel can come to your place of business or home with government officials and force you and your family members to take the vaccine ordered by the CDC. If at that time, you still refuse the injection, you will be considered a health risk to others and will be placed under arrest and quarantined at a government-operated facility. You will remain there until you submit to the injection or for a defined period of time. Once the pandemic is over, you will be released back into society.

You're probably in shock now in learning of this information and are probably saying to yourself, "this could never happen here in the land of the free." I pray it never happens either, but a similar situation erupted with one of our neighboring countries, Cuba, back in the early 1980s, when the mysterious outbreak of the HIV/AIDS virus started to show its head in every corner of the world. Its presence was identified first in Africa and the South Saharan Desert Regions. Cuba, a Communist country run by a dictator with the name of Fidel Castro, decided it was in the best interest of the country to isolate this disease as quickly as possible to prevent it from wiping out the entire population. A little eccentric, but his beliefs were not far-fetched. So Castro imposed martial law and forced every citizen in this Communist country to submit to an HIV test. In fact, by resisting his orders, citizens were not allowed to retain employment, get or keep their driver's license, or attend any educational institution. Self-quarantine was made law and enforced rigorously. The people who finally submitted to testing and received a negative test result lost the same freedoms they had prior to testing, meaning the right to privacy. Those who tested positive to the virus were taken into custody and transferred to one of the many "health camps" built by the dictator for the purpose of quarantining identified carriers of this incurable deadly disease.

Now it sounds worse than it was. The living conditions at these health camps were in many cases better than what the prisoners had in their normal lives. They received manual labor jobs, for which they received a salary. They also were allowed to send their earnings back home to their families. All medical care and treatment was provided to those who were in need of medical aid and their food and housing was free.

The prisoners only had to stay there as long as they were still testing positive for the HIV virus, and testing was conducted every three months. As soon as your test results reflected negative status and no viral loading was detectible in the blood test, you were free to leave and go home.

Fidel Castro's presidency ended in 2008, when Cuba's National Assembly chose his younger brother, Raul, to be the country's new president. Raul wrote a letter that was published in the state-run newspaper *Granma*. That's right, *Granma*. The letter clearly indicated that no changes to the existing confinement laws for HIV carriers would be adopted. Could that actually happen here in this country? Only the inevitable catastrophic events of the future will decide that. I am speaking of the next great plague.

Leading into this next segment, I will give you some sense of security and resolve as to the success researchers strive to achieve every day with the discovery and development of newer, safer, and more effective vaccinations. Let me first answer a few of the questions that are presented to me during my speaking engagements.

My audience is often confused as to the definition or difference between immunizations and inoculations. The role immunizations play is "to render immune." Immunizations protect susceptible patients from communicable (community) diseases by administering a living modified agent, such as Yellow Fever; a suspension of killed organisms like Pertussis; or a protein expressed in heterologous organisms, as with Hepatitis B Vaccines. Inoculations, or to inoculate, is the act of introducing a serum, vaccine, or antigen substance into a body. There is no doubt that vaccines play a major role in protecting many who choose to take them. Without vaccines, people who have weakened immune systems or are infected with a disease that compromises their immune system would be overwhelmed, leading to serious illness or death.

The reason the American Academy of Pediatric Medicine takes such a firm stance with its recommendations for infant and childhood vaccinations is that we know as the child approaches the age of three yrs, his or her body's own immune system starts to fully develop, rejecting and getting rid of the immunity given by the mother. This is when the immune system is at its weakest point, without the ability to respond and fight off disease. In the same way, the elderly (sixty years and above) have started to lose the viability and strength of their immune system. Everything changes with age!

Individuals who fit these criteria would benefit from vaccinations. The substance injected into their body is designed to fool the body into thinking it has just been invaded by an enemy and attack it before it makes the person sick, disabled, or dead. The body has millions and millions of scavenger cells in it that are always looking for these enemies. Once the genetic message is received by your immune system, it will create antibodies that will go out through your bloodstream and seek out and destroy those microbes. Mission accomplished!

The downsides to vaccines, just like with any drug, are their side effects. If you have been watching any TV lately, it seems as though every medical condition is being defined as a disease. We are bombarded with commercials peddling a new drug, vaccination, or supplement that says it will treat or cure your condition. These messages can be confusing and misleading. If the condition is due to a viral infection, remember that there are no cures for any virus ever discovered in science. However, viruses can be treated quickly and effectively. Bacterial infections are more difficult to treat but are curable. If you go to your physician and he or she diagnoses you with a viral infection and tells you, "Don't worry; I'll cure you," he or she is lying to you. Once your body has been invaded by a virus, you will have it for the rest of your life. You may have only one episode of illness and may not be infectious to anyone else, but you will be a carrier forever. If that same physician diagnoses you with a bacterial infection and claims he or she can cure you, remember that bacterial infections are curable but more difficult to treat.

Viruses are among the smallest microbes on earth, much smaller than bacteria. Viruses are not cells. They consist of only one or more molecules of DNA or RNA, which contain the virus's genes. If you were to look under a microscope, these viruses would look like tadpoles. Unlike most bacteria, viruses cause disease because they invade living healthy cells. Most viruses survive by taking over the genetic material that makes a cell work. When the virus sees a cell it likes, it attaches itself to the surface, called a receptor site, and then proceeds to inject molecules into the cell, such as DNA or RNA, and directs the cell to make new virus offspring, similar to sperm entering a fertile egg to create a fetus.

Microbes that belong to the bacteria group are made up of only one cell. Under a microscope, bacteria look like balls, rods, or spirals. Bacteria are so small that a line of one thousand could fit across the head of an eraser. And if you think that's small, you could fit one billion viruses across the same surface. Bacteria prefer mild temperatures like the human body and need oxygen to survive. But some bacteria can adapt to new environments and don't need any oxygen.

Depending then on the premise you have been infected with a virus, understand that the vaccine you were given years ago in your infancy or as a young child may have dissipated. The antibody levels may not be sufficient enough to protect you any longer. You may need to be revaccinated. Typically when you receive an injection, the side effects are isolated to just the injection site. This could present itself as redness, tenderness, or minor swelling and may be warm to the touch. If the symptoms you experience are more severe than this, you may be having an adverse or allergic reaction to that substance. If it becomes systemic, meaning affecting negatively other body systems, you may need to seek medical advice or treatment to counter the reaction.

Since the FDA requires full disclosure of any and all side effects that could occur with the advertised product, the manufacturer must include this information in literature and announcements on television commercials and provide consumers access to any documentation of these findings.

The side effects read like a rap sheet of a felon. With every vaccine, there are success stories and, of course, failures. On occasion, a vaccine may not work for the person injected. It wasn't recognized by his or her immune system, and therefore antibodies were never created. The body could also just simply reject it completely. The body will not keep what it doesn't recognize or need. Just like a vitamin, if you don't need it, the body gets rid of it.

With some vaccinations, you get a second chance for success. As an example, if you receive the three shots required for the Hepatitis B virus, which is the protocol, and then submit to the titer test (a simple blood test) and the results indicate antibody levels insufficient to protect you, your vaccinator can give you a fourth and final injection.

After reviewing the standard vaccination program approved by the American Academy of Pediatrics, backed by individual state immunization laws, I have compiled a complete list of the required vaccinations a person should receive based on a few criteria: the age of the person, current medical status, history of allergies, adverse reactions or complications documented with other injections, and travel plans. The reason I include future travels is because some destinations around the world may be experiencing a current outbreak of a particular disease or have a high concentration of infected people in that region with a particular illness.

There is a recommended immunization schedule for children aged zero through six years. If for any reason your child falls behind or starts late, the CDC has developed and approved a catch-up schedule. You can refer to the CDC website for a list of the recommended adult immunization schedule, United States 2011 (www.CDC.gov).

In addition to this formal version of the optimum vaccine schedule, there are alternative schedules, which include combination vaccines that stimulate an immune response much more quickly so you don't have to wait months for the immunization to work. The scientific and medical research communities worldwide have collaborated together in developing safer, more effective combination vaccines that reduce the number of doctor's visits, number of injections, and costs. With twelve separate vaccines on the childhood schedule and as many as six injections at any one visit, these combo vaccines will reduce the apprehension and phobias some children experience with injections.

The following is a list of the combination vaccines currently available:

- Chickenpox and Measles, Mumps, Rubella (MMR), combined as Proquad, made by Merck.
- DTaP, Hep B, and Polio, combined as Pediarix, made by GlaxcoSmithKline.
- Hib and Hep B, combined as Comvax, made by Merck.

- DTaP and Hib, combined as Trihibit, made by GlaxcoSmithKline. This can only be combined for the eighteen-month dose.
- Hep A and Hep B, combined as Twinrix, made by GlaxcoSmithKline. This may be given only to adults eighteen and older.
- DTaP-IPV, Hib, and Polio combined as Pentacel, made by GlaxcoSmithKline.
- DTaP and polio, combined as Kinrix, made by GlaxcoSmithKline.

The last two new combo vaccines are approved for use on children at two months, four months, and six months and adults eighteen years or older. If your child has already started the single-shot dose, he or she may continue with the combo vaccine. Just make sure the child hasn't received more than three polio injections in infancy.

So as you can see, there are many options that you and your infant or child have when it comes to immunizations. But like all drugs, there comes a price in the form of possible adverse reactions, allergic reactions, and medical side effects. After educating myself of the potential side effects that are associated with all vaccines, what I have concluded is that the majority of adverse reactions are usually isolated to the injection site. If you compare that to the side effects of drugs designed to treat infections, I begin to feel more comfortable in my decision making. With prescribed drugs, the list of side effects is so long, I often forget what the drug was originally designed to do for my condition to begin with.

Many drugs simply fail to work, exacerbate the symptoms, and cause disabling conditions or even death. Immunizations, on the other hand, can activate a dormant or latent disease already in your system or can create a large range of long-term chronic diseases and degenerative conditions. If you receive too many vaccines at the same time, this may cause the immune system to weaken by overwhelming it with antigens that exceed your body's response capabilities. It also may cause other conditions, such as Diabetes, Asthma, Autism, or Multiple Sclerosis to name a few.

The CDC and the FDA have deployed a post-licensure safety monitoring system that will keep reports and records of reported side effects of any particular drug, vaccine, supplement, or food product. Well, that gives me the "warm fuzzies," knowing that one government agency is collaborating with another to ensure public safety with these approved products. Imagine that—both agencies doing the checks and balances for the other. How convenient! I see a conflict of interest here.

Moving on, one cannot overlook the fact that the cons outweigh the pros for drugs and the pros outweigh the cons with vaccines.

The most controversial vaccine that changes every year is Influenza or the flu shot. Since a new type of Influenza is discovered every year, a new vaccine must be developed to give immunity for that particular strain, usually for life. Vaccines for the years 2010 to 2011 influenza season contained the following strains:

- A/California/7/09 H1N1-like virus
- A/Perth/16/2009 H3M2-like virus
- B/Brisbane/60-2008-like virus

There are three different types of Influenza: Type A, Type B, and Type C.

The CDC's Morbidity and Mortality Weekly Report (MMWR) identifies Influenza A viruses as annual epidemics, derived from different sources, such as humans, swine (pigs), and avian (bird). There have been sporadic cases of transmission of Influenza Viruses between humans and animals. According to a news release by the FDA in July 2010, they estimated 5 to 20 percent of the US population develops Influenza each year. This leads to more than

200 thousand hospitalizations from related complications and about thirty-six thousand deaths annually. These statistics provide some credence for the existing voluntary immunization program. Some notable Influenza epidemics from the past included Avian (H5N1 and H7N7) and Swine Influenza Viruses (H1N1, H1N2, and H3N2).

Influenza Type B is part of the genus family of viruses. Its host is only a single source, which are humans. Often referred to as "the flu," it is airborne and resides in the nose, throat, and lungs of the carrier. Influenza Type C is also part of the genus family and has one host, the human. The way you differentiate between B and C is by identifying its genetic makeup. Each consists of RNA that contains surface proteins called Hemagglutinin (H) and Neuraminidase (N). By looking through a microscope, we can identify the numbers of surface proteins, such as H1N1.

Once we discover the makeup, a vaccine is developed to fight the virus. The disease process for influenza works like this: A person is exposed to the virus through breathing, and it enters the bloodstream through mucous membranes that line the nose, throat, and airway. The host's immune system develops antibodies against the virus. As the virus changes or mutates, the first antibodies will no longer recognize the newer virus until the illness is well on its way. The symptoms typically experienced with infections are fever, coughing, headaches, and feeling tired or lethargic. Some carriers may progress to sore throats, nausea, vomiting, diarrhea, and fever. These symptoms can last from just a few days to a couple of weeks. With rare cases, the infected host may develop serious respiratory ailments that may require hospitalization. Death rarely occurs unless you have been exposed to a combination of different strains at the same time.

These symptoms are the same byproduct as from vaccines. However, the vaccine is typically given to high-risk individuals, such as the elderly (fifty-five years and older), children (newborn to age six), and those with weakened immune systems, such as HIV patients. In a news release, the FDA states, "There is always a possibility of a less optimal match between the virus strains that end up causing the most illness. However, even if the vaccine and the circulating strains are not an exact match, the vaccine may reduce the severity of the illness or may help prevent influenza-related complications." In my opinion, nothing in that statement indicates preventive medicine.

One manufacturer of the Influenza Virus Vaccine, CSL Limited, has been ordered by the FDA to conduct a study of Afluria in children, after obtaining information that the vaccine was causing a high incidence of fever and febrile seizures. Any of you parents want to volunteer your child in this research?

Given all this information with flu shots, many individuals are choosing not to vaccinate and are avoiding the flu shots. Typically when you get the flu, the symptoms are mild and tolerable, lasting just a few days and then you begin to feel better without a reoccurring bout with illness. More than likely, you have developed an immunity to the annual flu going around and don't need the flu shot anyway. However, if you are the person who gets deathly ill, meaning the symptoms are worse than what I previously listed and last longer than a few days, you could benefit from the flu shot. Statistics show that more people require hospitalization and die from complications from the flu shots than the number who expire from the natural flu every year. So now it's up to you to make that decision whether to continue to receive the vaccine or not.

The Hepatitis A vaccination after just one dose creates a successful immunity up to ninety-four percent on average but when followed with the second dose, the protection factor increases to 98.5 percent. Side effects reported are a sore arm that lasts a couple of days, with a small percentage reporting loss of appetite, low-grade fever, or tiredness.

The Hepatitis B vaccine is genetically engineered (man-made) and is

95 percent effective. It has been in use for the last twenty years, which is how long immunity is known to last and may last a lifetime. About 3 percent of those immunized experienced side effects, typically pain or tenderness around the injection site. Serious effects occur .001 percent of the time, usually a drug reaction (allergic reaction). No deaths have been recorded since its inception, so it has demonstrated its own merits to be one of the safest vaccines on the market.

Measles, Mumps, Rubella (MMR) has been thoroughly studied and tested in clinical trials; in combination with documented reports from recipients, it is claimed the only side effects are temporary and mild. The typical side effects that occur in less than 5 percent of patients were temporary joint pain, mild-grade fever, and mild rash. The overall protection factor runs an average of 90 percent or greater after two doses.

DTaP Vaccines have demonstrated a success rate of 98 percent or greater. Reports of severe side effects occur in less than one in every one million doses given—so rare, in fact, that it is difficult to determine if the vaccine was the root cause. Side effects have been reported as mild (fussiness)—good luck with that one if you are vaccinating a young child. Also reported were tiredness, fatigue, nausea, and occasional association with vomiting. Moderate problems could be nonstop crying (good luck with that one also) and mild-grade fever.

Typhoid Vaccine (inactivated) has reported side effects of fever, headache, redness or swelling, abdominal discomfort, nausea or vomiting, and rash with a small percentage of patients.

Varicella (Chickenpox)—Getting the Chicken Pox Vaccine is much safer than getting the Chickenpox disease. Most people receiving the vaccine do not have any problems with it. If any reactions occur, they are most likely after the first dose than after the second. Mild problems could include soreness or swelling where the shot was given; fever or rash has also been reported. The success or protection factor is 72 percent according to National Network for Immunization Information.

Yellow Fever—I think the name of the vaccine speaks for the side effects. This was given to me when I was being deployed for the Iraqi War in 1990. I received six other vaccines the same day, so it's impossible for me to indicate which vaccine caused the side effects I experienced, which were soreness around the injection sites and fever that lasted two days. The most common side effect with the

Yellow Fever vaccination is a moderate to high fever. Life-threatening severe illness has occurred with about one person in every 250,000. This last problem can lead to organ failure and death. However, that has never been reported with the booster shot. The protection factor stated by National Network for Immunization Information is 95 percent and last approximately 10 years or possibly a life time with some.

Meningococcal vaccine has a history of mild side effects that occur in nearly half the people who get the injection. The problems reported are redness or pain around the injection site and/or fever. A serious nervous system disorder, called Guillain-Barre Syndrome (or GBS), has been reported among some people. The percentage is not indicated because of the possibility of delayed hereditary involvement. The reported protection factor as of April 2010, by the National Network for Immunization Information is between 85 – 100 percent.

Tetanus is given to provide protection (immunity) against "lockjaw." Side effects may occur in a small percentage of patients, who reported mild fever, muscle aches, tiredness, nausea, itching and swelling near the injection site, and rash. The medication is administered into a muscle, not a vein or artery. The Tetanus Vaccine has a protection factor of approximately 100 percent and should last up to ten years after vaccination.

HPV, the vaccine to prevent cervical cancer, has recently come under great scrutiny by both the public and the medical community as a whole. What was thought to prevent cervical cancer may actually do the opposite. The side effects also are many. These include redness and swelling around the injection site, high fever, headaches, fatigue, nausea and vomiting, fainting episodes, loss of appetite, severe abdominal pain, muscle joint pain, jerking movements, dizziness, vision changes, and ringing in the ears. Need I go any further?

The risks of side effects with the HPV Vaccine and complications that go along with it clearly outweigh the benefits, which have yet to be determined. More human research must occur to determine accurate information of its benefits versus its side effects, including the possible development of cervical cancer. I give this one a thumbs-down. But you may still want to consult your doctor and get a second or third or fourth opinion.

My investigation led me to discover that the pharmaceutical companies, vaccine manufacturers, and FDA fail to conduct enough research as to the potential impact the vaccines could have on both the disease and the patient. They also fail to collect accurate statistics and deny any long-term side effects that may occur with the products. Basic testing for the results of base line blood levels and comparison test results after vaccinating is rarely conducted. The primary reason the the FDA doesn't insist on more extensive human research is because it has ruled "heal prick samples" are to invasive.

The FDA over looks its most basic function, which is to help Americans identify and protect themselves from potentially dangerous substances. Much of the research is kept confidential and is released to individuals on a need-to-know basis only. The majority of the research done today is on controlled groups, volunteers (usually foreign prisoners and animals). On rare occasions human test models have volunteered their bodies for the purpose of research and development.

Human Right Groups and conspiracy believers have tried to make a connection between human cleansing and vaccine research.

The bottom line is that, as you can see, when you or your child is vaccinate, there always exist a chance of side effects. What I have learned through a lot of research is that the manufacturers and providers of these vaccines are protected from any liability in civil court and federal vaccine injury compensation is very difficult to get.

Why not just throw a little salt on the injection site? No pharmaceutical company or manufacturer will claim that their vaccine will, 100 percent of the time, protect you from infection. If I understand this correctly so far, it appears you are giving permission to the attending physician to inject a drug into your or your child's body to protect from an infection or disease you may never be exposed to. Also, by accepting the vaccine, you may be predisposing you or your child to the side effects that some of these vaccines have been documented to cause. I think I just came up with a new business concept. It's called "vaccine insurance." Don't let anyone force your child to take a vaccine without your voluntary, informed consent.

If a doctor threatens you, or refuses to provide treatment to you or your child on the grounds that you refuse to be vaccinated, find another doctor and report the situation to the state medical board. It is against the law for any licensed medical practitioner to withhold treatment to anyone on the grounds that he or she refused vaccination. If a doctor or government official denies a medical or religious exemption that you have filed with the courts, get an attorney to advise you what actions may be taken against them legally.

In closing, I hope you have gained a better perspective of how important the role of preventive medicine and immunity are to help you with breaking the chain of disease.

Chapter 9
Our Future Existence In
This Microbial World

The last question that remains to be answered is: What is going to happen to the human race with predictions of great plagues and pandemics just over the horizon? The entire context of this book has taken you on a journey to help you understand the impact these outbreaks of disease and illness have on all of us. We have discovered that, despite recent breakthroughs with new types of drugs, immunizations, treatments and therapies, screening and testing techniques, early detection systems, and public awareness, little has been done to stop these catastrophic disease events from occurring. Unfortunately, human bodies, unlike any other life-form on earth, are very vulnerable to these enemies. They can intrude in our lives at any given moment.

The human body, however, is extremely resilient, with a unique self-defense system. Our bodies have a network of protective mechanisms not found in other living species. We are covered with a shield of armor (skin), which is impenetrable when intact, and we have an immune system made up of billions of fighting warriors that won't stop fighting these invaders until their death. So why do I feel like the under card in a UFL (ultimate fighting league) event? These microbes carry an arsenal of weapons that can penetrate all of our defense mechanisms without detection.

Seemingly without warning, a new strain or mutation of a preexisting disease appears again, only to wreak more havoc with the human species once again. It's like a football team you just played against last season, and all they did was change their jersey. The predictions for our future in this world filled with microbes appear on the surface to be more of a scare tactic than reality. The media has a lot to do with this. For a few decades now, these events have made great news headlines. I refer to this as Popular Media Pandemic (PMP). It's a syndrome that is more devastating than the disease itself. There have been numerous news articles, documentaries, and books all with one mission in mind, to create interest that leads to panic and then fear. This book simply brought to your attention risk factors that you can change in your own life through awareness and a resolve that can break the chain of disease, all disease.

Some of these titles alone give me the sense of hopelessness. Do you remember *The Andromeda Strain*, a 1969 novel authored by Michael Crichton (science fiction); *Company of Liars* by Karen Maitland in 2008 (speculation and theory); *The Last Canadian* in 1974 by William Heine; *The Last Town on Earth* in 2006 by Thomas Mullen; *The Stand* in 1978 by Stephen King (a great storyteller); *World War Z* in 2006 by Max Brooks (misguided reality); and *Doomsday Book* in 1992 by Connie Willis (need I say more?—I'm still here to read it)?

The films produced depicting the inevitable demise of the human race as we know it also can take credit for taking what is a serious health issue and simply making it entertaining. There is nothing criminal about that; even I like a good thriller once in a while. I was only two years old at the time the classic movie *The Last Man Standing* came out in 1964 (horror/science fiction), based on the novel *I Am Legend* by Richard Matheson. Who could forget the film classic *Twelve*

Monkeys, which came out in 1995, based on the story of a future world devastated by disease? My favorite to date is *Outbreak*, from 1995. This film focused on an outbreak of a fictional Ebola-like virus called Motaba in Zaire, which shows up in a small town in the United States. The fictional horror film *28 Days Later*, in 2002, depicted the outbreak of an infectious "rage" virus that destroys all of mainland Britain. The three most current films in this category are *Doomsday* (2008), *After Armageddon* (2010), and finally, one I have yet to see, *Contagion* (2011).

In reality, the next great plague will happen in one of two ways, either natural or man-made bioterrorism. Both of these events will be extremely difficult if not impossible to prevent. However, with adequate preparation and early detection and reporting, we could limit the devastation these events could have on civilization as a whole. This is a global undertaking that will need cooperation and collaboration from every nation.

If these events were to occur naturally, there are a number of ways that could jump-start a global pandemic. These are just some examples of the scenarios that could play out:

- Extreme climate changes and ecological imbalance
- World population and agricultural crisis
- Supervolcano
- Megatsunami
- Meteorite impact or other cosmic events

If the event were to occur as a result of man-made terrorism, there are numerous ways to infuse these microbes into society. A couple of years back; I authored a curriculum for the Office of Homeland Security that was titled "Bioterrorist Pandemic Preparedness." The events described in the training element such as a bioterrorist infused microbe, remains as a real-life risk to every person residing within our borders and around the world. According to the Centers for Disease

Control and Prevention (CDC), the definition of a bioterrorist attack is the deliberate release of viruses, bacteria, toxins, or other harmful agents used to cause illness or death in people. These agents are usually found in nature, and it is possible because of genetic engineering to alter or change their ability to cause harm. These agents also can be manufactured in such a way as to make them resistant to vaccines and medicines. Biological agents can be spread through the air, water, and agricultural products. Terrorists prefer these agents because they are difficult to detect and do not cause illness for several hours or days.

When I was first approached with developing a plan for law enforcement agencies to use with the goal of defending against such attacks, the model I used was the water supply source for the entire city of San Francisco. What I discovered in my research was how vulnerable that region was to a bioterrorist attack. It turned out that the Hetch Hetchy Dam is the primary source of water for the San Francisco Bay area. The canal is gravity fed, so no pumping stations were constructed. There are agents that could be infused into the water supply there that would potentially cause illness or death to the entire populace. The poison could be Typhoid, Botulism, or Salmonella.

In Oregon in 1984, there was an attempt to control a local election by incapacitating the local population. By accomplishing this, the majority of voters became ill and with many requiring hospitalization, preventing them from voting. This was done by infecting salad bars in eleven restaurants, produce in the grocery stores, doorknobs, and other public facilities with Salmonella Bacteria. The attack was linked to 751 people becoming ill; however, there were no fatalities.

If the organism were airborne, people who inhaled an infectious aerosol would generally experience severe respiratory illness, including life-threatening pneumonia and systemic infection.

Today, the CDC and WHO are composing a list to identify the most threatening pandemics based on faults in critical areas of identification of the microbe, our ability to isolate it from spreading from the host locale, reliable means for treating the illness (antibiotics), and testing procedures to identify newly infected patients. The current list of names or types of microorganisms that pose the greatest health today includes:

- Viral hemorrhagic fevers
- Antibiotic-resistant pathogens
- SARS
- Influenza H5N1

The Centers for Disease Control and Prevention built labs and research chambers in Atlanta, Georgia, that house the deadliest types of microbes and pathogens ever discovered on the face of the earth. The BL4 chamber, which stands for biological level 4, contains viruses, bacteria, and an arsenal of microbes that currently have no cure or vaccine.

These chambers house the Congo Virus, Crimean Hemorrhagic Fever Virus, Dengue Fever Virus, Equine Encephalitis Eirus, Ebola Virus, Hantavirus, Lassa Virus, Marburg, Monkeypox, Tick-borne Encephalitis, Whitepox, and Yellow Fever. Most of these particle viruses erupt in stages in isolated villages. Many conspiracy believers put the blame on CDC researchers and only a handful of others are allowed into these regions. Their belief is that the US government has created genetically altered viruses and intentionally released them into these small, unsuspecting villages, which have little or no access to medical care and no government to protect them. After the outbreak has been reported, our scientists go into the infected area to get a body count of the sick, dying, and dead. They record the symptomatic stages, isolate the virus, and leave the site, usually within twenty-four hrs. The pathogen is then returned to the United States and stored in the two BL4 chambers located in Atlanta Georgia and at

CDC Headquarters in Washington D.C. can handle this level of microorganism existence.

Back at the original site, those villagers who have not succumbed to the effects of the disease process are given rations and medical supplies that will sustain them for forty-eight hours. In addition, they are given specific directions of how they are to dispose of the dead. Remember that we have no information about these mysterious diseases and don't know how they are transmitted from host to host. We also don't know if they are related to other life-forms like monkeys or apes or a food source or water. These researchers and scientist have not identified its viability in the environment, or stability outside the human body. For this reason you can't just bury the bodies; you must incinerate them and burn all objects they may have come in contact with. I am writing this with as much compassion as possible and with an unbiased approach. What really occurs is far more devastating. Typically the researchers and their support staff burn the entire village down, leaving no evidence of the microorganism's presence.

The other categories of pathogens that are contained in these chambers are: Rickettsiae, Bacteria, Toxins, Fungi, Ricin (D and E) and Saxitoxins.

The reason for not listing these organisms by their biological name was to avoid boring you with pages of scientific information that will do nothing in your quest to lead a disease-free life. Just remember the term "universal precautions."

Now back to the research part of this scenario. Prior to the scientists entering the BL4 chamber, they first must put on a cut-resistant bodysuit complete with hand gloves, booties, and headgear that has been stitched together and taped. No skin is exposed to the outside world. They also wear chemical and radiation sensors and are provided air and oxygen that has been purified and filtered for any microorganisms. They enter through a system of double doors that open and close themselves. Any air leaving the chamber goes through twelve filtration stations before being sent back to the atmosphere. These precautionary procedures are necessary to maintain the most sterile environments possible. This, however, is not feasible with emergency departments or operating facilities.

The immediate concern is the sudden and unexpected appearance of a hemorrhagic fever virus. These types and subtypes of viruses are usually resistant to the most effective antiviral agents currently available and are acute illnesses (physical symptoms erupt quickly). Furthermore, mortality rates are among the highest of the viral families. Once symptoms begin (usually within twenty-four to forty-eight hours after exposure), the virus excels in producing numbers our immune response can't keep up with. Flulike symptoms become more severe to the point that the fevers are so high (106° F and higher) the bodily systems and organs begin to shut down and hemorrhage. You literally hemorrhage (bleed to death). There have been dozens of types of hemorrhagic viruses discovered around the world, but the most prevalent and deadly are Dengue, Marburg, Ebola, and Hanta (respiratory) virus.

The well-known Salmonella Virus could have the same impact. Here is a case scenario: One day an expectant mother in her thirties goes to her doctor's office complaining of severe stomach pain, vomiting, diarrhea, fever, and chills. It appears on the surface to be directly related to the pregnancy. The expectant mother is given IV fluids and a prescription for Fluoroquinolone—an antibiotic—and is sent home. The woman later has a miscarriage, followed by her own death.

The next day, a two-year-old boy is presented in an emergency room in Massachusetts complaining of the same symptoms. He is also given an IV of fluids and administered Cephalosporin (an antibiotic). The boy's lab results come back positive for salmonella, a common food-borne bacterial infection, but in his case, the bacteria are super-resistant to antibiotics. The boy dies of dehydration and bloodstream infection.

What most of the public isn't aware of is that once you exhaust the supply of drugs approved to control or destroy these "super bugs," the body tries to protect itself by naturally shunting water to the area infected. The number one leading cause of death in the world every year is dehydration (lack of fluids) and malnutrition (lack of nutrients). These two conditions kill more people than all other diseases combined, according to the World Health Organization.

A couple of days later, the infection spreads, causing the death toll to rise to 325, with thousands of children, the elderly, and other vulnerable individuals packing emergency rooms across the Northeast, all complaining of similar symptoms. Cases are now being reported in fifteen states along the East Coast, with isolated cases reported in California and Texas. Mexico is now reporting fourteen cases and Canada twenty-seven cases.

The next day, reports put the death toll at 1730, with 220,000 cases. The epidemic spreads to other counties via international air travel. Canada, Mexico, and Europe close their borders to US food imports, and travel initiated in the United States is banned around the globe. The economic impact cripples the United States and other countries, soon reaching tens of billions of dollars. The FDA and CDC identify the source of the outbreak as contaminated milk from a distribution center in New York State.

Think this scenario can't happen? Think again. This same scenario occurred in 1985 and infected 200,000 people in the Midwest.

The next disease on our list of potential pandemics that may occur this century—I will say next year for a sense of urgency—is severe acute respiratory syndrome (SARS). This is a virus that results in a severe respiratory ailment that has a 10 percent fatality rate. SARS, which is a member of the Coronavirus, first emerged in 2002 and

2003 in the city of Hong Kong. Hong Kong alone was considered a pandemic zone. There were 8422 cases that resulted in 916 deaths. Eventually, there were cases reported in thirty-seven countries by early 2003. As of 2011, the spread of SARS has been fully contained, with only one case reported from a laboratory-induced infection in China. SARS, however, has not been eradicated (unlike smallpox) because of its presence in its natural host (animal populations).

This epidemic reached the public spotlight in 2003, when an American businessman traveling from China became inflicted with pneumonia-like symptoms while on a flight from Singapore. The plane stopped in Vietnam, where the victim later died. Many of the medical staff who treated him also became infected with the virus, including an Italian doctor who died shortly after reporting the case to the World Health Organization (WHO).

On March 13, 2003, WHO issued a global alert, followed by a health alert by the CDC. The lack of reporting this information more quickly to the people of China caused concerned citizens in Hong Kong to create a website www.sosick.org. The interaction and contact that farmers have with their livestock could lead to another outbreak in the future. No vaccine has been developed to date.

The next disease in our future is the Influenza Virus H5N1. Also known as the "bird flu," it is a subtype of influenza A. This virus, which causes illness in humans and many other animal species, is a highly pathogenic avian influenza. The recent outbreak in 2006 to 2007 appeared in Asia and killed tens of millions of birds and spurred the slaughter of hundreds of millions more to stop its spread. The H5N1 avian (bird) flu is continuing to gradually grow in epidemic areas, but is being held in check in bird farms by vaccination. The global situation with H5N1 hasn't changed much since those outbreaks. Reports of infected humans usually occur when farmers come in contact with infected birds and the surfaces that have been contaminated with secretions or excretions. Some genetic parts of current human influenza A viruses had their origin with infected birds. Influenza A viruses are constantly changing, and over time they again may adapt to the human host. So how does influenza type A bird flu that infected a human begin to globe-trot around? There are numerous avenues, such as international travel, human trafficking (Asian bride anyone?), and imported poultry that is infected with the virus.

These outbreaks have now been reported by WHO in Asia and parts of Europe, the Near East, and Africa, with a mortality rate about 60 percent of those reported infected. Scientists remain concerned that HPAI H5N1 viruses have the potential to possibly change into a form that is able to spread easily from person to person. There are two vaccines approved by the US Food and Drug Administration, but they are not recommended for treatment at this time because of the possibility that the virus will become drug-resistant. The message I get from the deliberate withholding of a successful vaccine that could save potentially thousands of lives and *might* lead to drug resistance is a blatant disregard for human life.

These scenarios are not your fault. You have gained critical information on ways you and your family can identify these situations, prevent exposure, protect yourselves under all circumstances, and most importantly break the chain of transmission. The entities that have been put in place with taxpayer money and supported by special interest groups like the pharmaceutical companies have dropped the ball with their promise to protect us, the people of the United States. The Centers for Disease Control and *Prevention* (CDC), National Institutes of Health (NIH), and National Institute of Allergy and Infectious Diseases (NIAID) have been investigated by the Infectious Diseases Society of America (IDSA) for what could be viewed as research and development (R&D) malpractice.

About 2 million people acquire bacterial infections just in US hospitals every year, and 90,000 die as a result, according to the

CDC. About 70 percent of those infections were resistant to at least one drug. The trends toward increasing numbers of infections and increasing drug resistance show no signs of abating. The end result is a $5 billion annual burden placed on U.S. citizens. The pipeline of new antibiotics is drying up. The major pharmaceutical companies have lost interest with developing new antibiotics because these drugs simply are not as profitable as drugs that treat chronic (long-term) conditions. You know the old saying: If the engine never breaks, we won't need mechanics.

Drug R&D is expensive, risky, and time-consuming. Most drug programs require ten years of research and an investment of $800 million to $1.7 billion to bring to market. These figures are reflective in the FDA Fiscal Accountability Report. The pharmaceutical companies know that their industry impacts every single human being in the world. No other industries have the same control over our health and lives. People are willing in many cases to pay whatever it takes to protect themselves from disease (immunizations), solve their aches and pains (drugs), and prolong their sanity and health as they grow older (drugs, pain supplements, and psycho-meds).

The controversy of tapping into this power is simply motivated by greed. Some of the Chief Executives, Chief Operations Officers, and Chief Financial Officers of these conglomerates have changed their titles and names and sit on the steering and approval committees of the FDA. In a sense, they are approving their own drugs to go to market. Conspiracy theory? Not quite! This recently caught the eyes of watchdog groups and was uncovered during Congressional hearings, and was broadcast on the news heard in the United States.

So what are we faced with in the coming months or years with these patent-pending outbreaks (pandemics)? Only the future will tell. You, however, don't have to sit around and wait for these health-related events to impact you and make you the next statistic. Use the tools and resources I've presented to you in this book and decrease your odds of becoming the next victim. These catastrophic events could start with one person sitting next to you in a movie theater, standing next to you in an elevator, eating from the same salad bar as you, working out on the weight machine at your local health club, coughing and sneezing in the checkout line at the grocery store, or someone you're intimate with.

Remember, it simply takes breaking just one of those four links and you could lead a disease-free life. The chain of protection I've laid out for you is simple:

- Avoid contact with a potentially or known infectious person (have them get tested if concerned of their status).
- Assume that all body fluids and secretions contain a transmittable disease in them (universal precautions).
- Protect any disruption in the continuity of your skin with proper first aid materials.
- Utilize personal protective equipment when engaged in sexual behavior and while performing professional tasks.
- Get tested routinely to identify if you have been infected (screening and testing).

If you follow these guidelines, you will have taken the first steps to leading a disease-free life.

RICHARD F. DEROSE,

As an infectious disease specialist, Mr. DeRose, a global consultant based in Southern California, is a compassionate and dedicated individual who helps educate and protect people from the challenges and often frightening states we are exposed to daily.

Mr. DeRose's areas of expertise include infectious diseases, such as HIV, hepatitis, tuberculosis (TB), sexually transmitted disease (STD), and skin conditions related to MRSA. His extensive training focused on all kinds of infections, including those caused by bacteria, viruses, fungi, and parasites. In some ways, Mr. DeRose is like a medical detective—he examines difficult cases looking for clues to identify the culprit, and then he integrates the information into his public-speaking engagements.

As Mr. DeRose states, "I love being in the trenches practicing infectious disease management. Initially I was drawn to the attention that HIV/AIDS was receiving from the international media pools. That evolved into my passion for identifying other diseases of all kinds so I could help people protect themselves, take precautionary steps to avoid exposure, receive appropriate care, and then get on with their lives. My approach with all diseases is with respect and safety.

"Ignorance is not bliss.

"What you don't know will eventually harm you. I take great pride in providing the most accurate information and presenting it to my clients through sensitive and compassionate leadership."

ABOUT MR. DEROSE:

I wrote Breaking the Chain of Disease to rediscover the world of infectious diseases that impact every person on the face of the earth. The information will give you the history of disease, past, present and future. It will describe the social microbe factories that surround us in every environment. The book will update the reader as to the ever changing world of sexual behavior and promiscuity.

The information provided throughout this book will accurately demonstrate the chain of events that lead to the transmission of all diseases from one human host to another. The reader will learn the use of protective measures and good hygienic practices that will decrease their chances of infection.

You will discover that the Government Agencies, Pharmaceutical Companies and Medical providers mislead us with false hopes to cure or help treat the developing infections, epidemics and pandemics that develop around the globe.

This book is the perfect prescription to leading a healthier and disease free life.

www.ingramcontent.com/pod-product-compliance
Lightning Source LLC
Chambersburg PA
CBHW021955170526
45157CB00003B/1000